FORMULARY FOR
LABORATORY ANIMALS

FORMULARY FOR LABORATORY ANIMALS

COMPILED BY

C. TERRANCE HAWK, PhD, DVM, Dipl. ACLAM

AND

STEVEN L. LEARY, DVM, Dipl. ACLAM

IN ASSOCIATION WITH THE

AMERICAN COLLEGE OF

LABORATORY ANIMAL MEDICINE

IOWA STATE UNIVERSITY PRESS / AMES

C. TERRANCE HAWK received his PhD from the University of Arizona and his DVM from Purdue University School of Veterinary Medicine. He is presently Deputy Director and Head of Clinical Services, Division of Laboratory Animal Resources, Duke University Medical Center, Durham, North Carolina.

STEVEN L. LEARY received his DVM degree from Iowa State University College of Veterinary Medicine. He is presently Assistant Vice Chancellor for Veterinary Affairs, Division of Comparative Medicine, Washington University School of Medicine, St. Louis, Missouri.

© 1995 Iowa State University Press, Ames, Iowa 50014
All rights reserved

Authorization to photocopy items for internal or personal use, or the internal or personal use of specific clients, is granted by Iowa State University Press, provided that the base fee of $.10 per copy is paid directly to the Copyright Clearance Center, 27 Congress Street, Salem, MA 01970. For those organizations that have been granted a photocopy license by CCC, a separate system of payments has been arranged. The fee code for users of the Transactional Reporting Service is 0-8138-2422-2/95 $.10.

∞ Printed on acid-free paper in the United States of America

First edition, 1995

Library of Congress Cataloging-in-Publication Data

Hawk, C. Terrance
    Formulary for laboratory animals / compiled by C. Terrance Hawk and Steven L. Leary; in association with the American College of Laboratory Animal Medicine.—1st ed.
        p.   cm.
    Includes bibliographical references (p.   ).
    ISBN 0-8138-2422-2
    1. Veterinary drugs. 2. Veterinary drugs—Dosage. 3. Veterinary prescriptions. 4. Laboratory animals—Diseases—Chemotherapy. I. Leary, Steven L. II. American College of Laboratory Animal Medicine. III. Title.
SF917.H25   1995
636.089'514—dc20   95-23190

Last digit is the print number: 9 8 7 6 5 4 3 2

CONTENTS

PREFACE

$\mathcal{S}$EVERAL YEARS AGO WHILE
we were at the University of Alabama at Birmingham, it became
evident that a formulary for use in laboratory animal medicine
would be extremely useful. While there are many excellent references available, few contain a comprehensive list of drugs. This
formulary grew out of the need to make drug dosages available in
a single publication that can be carried in the coat pocket of the
laboratory animal veterinarian, and to also serve as a resource for
the private practitioner and the scientific investigator. It is our
hope that we have succeeded in our effort. Our intent is to con-
stantly collect drug dosages and other useful information to in-
clude in subsequent editions. With this in mind we solicit our
reader's input. All comments and suggestions to improve this
book will be appreciated. Send your comments to Dr. C.T. Hawk,
Division of Laboratory Animal Resources, Duke University
Medical Center, Box 3180, Durham, NC 27710-3180, or you
may send comments via electronic mail to Dr. Hawk:
thawk@acpub.duke.edu

The drug dosages listed in this formulary were derived from
hundreds of journals and textbooks. We recommend that the references be consulted to determine the circumstances under which
the stated dosages were used. We believe that professional judg-
ment is necessary to select the proper dose.

ABBREVIATIONS

Species

Am	Amphibians	**Fi**	Fish	**N**	Nonhuman primates
Bi	Birds	**G**	Gerbils	**Rb**	Rabbits
Bo	Bovine	**Go**	Goats	**Rc**	Raccoons
C	Cats	**Gp**	Guinea pigs	**R**	Rats
Ch	Chinchillas	**H**	Hamsters	**Re**	Reptiles
D	Dogs	**M**	Mice	**Sh**	Sheep
F	Ferrets	**Mi**	Mink	**Sw**	Swine

Dosages, Measures, and Methods

bid	twice daily	mg	milligrams
BW	body weight	ml	milliliters
d	day	mm	millimeters
g	grams	O/D	outside diameter
G	gauge	PO	by mouth (per os)
h	hours	prn	as needed
IA	intraarterially	q	every
IC	intracoelomically	qid	four times daily
IM	intramuscularly	qod	every other day
IP	intraperitoneally	SC	subcutaneously
IPP	intrapleuroperitoneally	sid	once daily
IT	intratracheally	tid	three times daily
IV	intravenously	Tbs	tablespoon (approximately 15 ml)
kg	kilograms	tsp	teaspoon (approximately 5 ml)
L	liters	u	units
lb	pounds	%	g/100 mls

FORMULARY

ANALGESICS AND SEDATIVES

Acepromazine

C   0.1-0.2 mg/kg BW IM, SC (Kinsell, 1986)
0.5-1.0 mg/lb BW PO prn (Kinsell, 1986)
D   0.1-0.5 mg/kg BW IV, IM, SC (Kinsell, 1986)
0.25-1.0 mg/lb BW PO prn (Kinsell, 1986)
F   0.2 mg/kg BW IM (Flecknell, 1987)
G   May precipitate seizures (Harkness and Wagner, 1983)
Go 0.05-0.5 mg/kg BW IM (Swindle and Adams, 1988)
0.55 mg/kg BW IV (Swindle and Adams, 1988)
0.05-0.1 mg/kg BW IM (NCSU, 1987)
M   1-2 mg/kg BW IM (Harkness and Wagner, 1983)
2-5 mg/kg BW IP (Flecknell, 1987)
N   0.5-1.0 mg/kg BW IM, SC (Melby and Altman, 1976)
0.2 mg/kg BW IM (Flecknell, 1987)
R   1-2 mg/kg BW IM (Harkness and Wagner, 1983)
Rb 1-2 mg/kg BW IM (Harkness and Wagner, 1983)
5 mg/kg BW IM (Flecknell, 1987)
2 mg/kg BW IM (Bauck, 1989)
Rc 2-2.5 mg/kg BW (Evans and Evans, 1986)
Re 0.125-0.5 mg/kg BW IM (Frye, 1981)
Sh 0.05-0.5 mg/kg BW IM (Swindle and Adams, 1988)
0.55 mg/kg BW IV (Swindle and Adams, 1988)
Sw 0.11-0.22 mg/kg BW SC, IM, IV (Swindle and Adams, 1988)
0.05-0.1 mg/kg BW IM (NCSU, 1987)
0.03-0.22 mg/kg BW IM not to exceed 15 mg total (NCSU, 1987)

Acetaminophen

D   15 mg/kg BW PO q8h (Jenkins, 1987)

M   300 mg/kg BW PO (Jenkins, 1987)
N   5-10 mg/kg BW PO (Johnson et al, 1981)
R   110-300 mg/kg BW PO (Jenkins, 1987)
        100-300 mg/kg BW PO q4h (Flecknell, 1991)

Acetaminophen and codeine

Rb   1 ml elixer/100 ml drinking water (Wixson, 1994)

Alphadolone/alphaxalone (Saffan)

C   9 mg/kg BW IM (Flecknell, 1987)
Gp   40 mg/kg BW IM (Flecknell, 1987)
N   12-18 mg/kg BW IM (Flecknell, 1987)
R   9-12 mg/kg BW IP (Flecknell, 1987)
Rb   9-12 mg/kg BW IM (Flecknell, 1987)
Sw   6 mg/kg BW IM (Flecknell, 1987)

Aminopyrine

D   265 mg total PO (Borchard et al, 1990)
Gp   130 mg/kg BW PO (Jenkins, 1987)
H   130 mg/kg BW PO (Jenkins, 1987)
M   150 mg/kg BW IP (Borchard et al, 1990)
        300 mg/kg BW PO (Borchard et al, 1990)
R   200 mg/kg BW SC (Borchard et al, 1990)
        650 mg total PO ((Borchard et al, 1990)
Rb   50 mg/kg BW PO (Jenkins, 1987)

Antipyrine

C   100 mg/kg BW IM, IP, SC (Borchard et al, 1990)
        500 mg/kg BW PO (Borchard et al, 1990)
D   1000 mg total PO (Borchard et al, 1990)
M   197 mg/kg BW IP (Borchard et al, 1990)
R   600 mg/kg BW SC (Borchard et al, 1990)
        220 mg/kg BW SC (Borchard et al, 1990)
Rb   100 mg/kg BW PO (Jenkins, 1987)
        100 mg/kg BW IM, IP, SC (Borchard et al, 1990)
        500 mg/kg BW PO (Borchard et al, 1990)

Aspirin

C 10 mg/kg BW PO q48h (Jenkins, 1987)
1 children's aspirin (1.25 gr) PO q36h (Kinsell, 1986)

D 10-20 mg/kg BW PO q12h (Jenkins, 1987)

Note: Use buffered tabs: analgesic dose 10 mg/kg BW PO q12h (Kinsell, 1986)
Antirheumatic maximum dose 40 mg/kg BW q18h (Kinsell, 1986)

Go 10-20 mg/kg BW PO (Swindle and Adams, 1988)

Gp 270 mg/kg BW IP sid (CCAC, 1984)
86 mg/kg BW PO, try q4h (Flecknell, 1987)

H 240 mg/kg BW IP sid (CCAC, 1984)

M 120-300 mg/kg BW PO (Jenkins, 1987)
120 mg/kg BW PO q4h (Flecknell, 1987)
400 mg/kg BW SC sid (CCAC, 1984)
25 mg/kg BW IP (Borchard et al, 1990)

N 100 mg/kg BW PO sid (CCAC, 1984)
20 mg/kg BW PO q6-8h (Flecknell, 1987)

R 100 mg/kg BW PO q4h (Jenkins, 1987; Flecknell, 1987)
400 mg/kg BW SC, PO (Harkness and Wagner, 1983)

Rb 400 mg/kg BW SC, PO sid (Harkness and Wagner, 1983)
100 mg/kg BW PO, try q4h (Flecknell, 1991)
20 mg/kg BW PO sid (equiv to 600 mg dose in humans) (Marangos et al, 1994)

Sh 10-20 mg/kg BW PO (Swindle and Adams, 1988)

Sw 10-20 mg/kg BW PO q4h (Swindle and Adams, 1988)

Buprenorphine

Bi 0.05 mg/kg BW SC, IM (Nemetz, 1990)

C 0.005-0.01 mg/kg BW SC, IM q12h (Jenkins, 1987; Flecknell, 1985)

D 0.01-0.02 mg/kg BW SC q12h (Jenkins, 1987; Flecknell, 1985)

G 0.1-0.2 mg/kg BW SC q8h (Flecknell, 1987)

Gp 0.05 mg/kg BW SC q8-12h (Jenkins, 1987; Flecknell, 1985)
0.05 mg/kg BW SC q6-12h (Flecknell, 1991)

H 0.05 mg/kg BW SC q8-12h (Jenkins, 1987)
0.5 mg/kg BW SC q8h (Flecknell, 1987)

M 2 mg/kg BW SC q12h (Jenkins, 1987; Flecknell, 1985)
2.5 mg/kg BW IP q6-8h (Jenkins, 1987)
0.05-0.1 mg/kg BW SC q6-12h (Flecknell, 1991)

N   0.01 mg/kg BW IM, IV q12h (Jenkins, 1987; Flecknell, 1985)
R   0.1-0.5 mg/kg BW SC, IV q12h (Jenkins, 1987; Flecknell, 1985; Flecknell, 1987)
    0.006 mg/ml drinking water (Deeb et al, 1989)
Rb 0.02-0.05 mg/kg BW SC, IM, IV q8-12h (Jenkins, 1987; Flecknell, 1985)
    0.01-0.05 mg/kg BW SC, IV q6-12h (Flecknell, 1991)
Sh 0.005-0.01 mg/kg BW IM q4-6h (Flecknell, 1989)
Sw 0.005-0.01 mg/kg BW IM, IV (Swindle and Adams, 1988)

Note: Up to 0.1 mg/kg BW can be used for major surgical procedures (Farris, 1990)

Butorphanol

C   0.4 mg/kg BW BW SC q6h (Jenkins, 1987)
D   0.2-0.4 mg/kg BW SC, IM, IV q2-5h (Jenkins, 1987)
M   0.05-5.0 mg/kg BW SC q4h (Jenkins, 1987)
    5.4 mg/kg BW SC (Wright, et al, 1985)
    1-5 mg/kg BW SC q4h (Flecknell, 1991)
R   0.05-2.0 mg/kg BW SC q4h (Jenkins, 1987)
    2 mg/kg BW SC q4h (Flecknell, 1991)
Rb 0.1-0.5 mg/kg BW IV q4h (Flecknell, 1989)
Sh 0.5 mg/kg BW SC q2-3h (Flecknell, 1989)
Sw 0.1-0.3 mg/kg BW IM (Swindle and Adams, 1988)

Chlorpromazine

C   1-2 mg/kg BW IV, IM q12h (Kinsell, 1986)
D   0.55-4.4 mg/kg BW IV q6-24h (Kinsell, 1986)
    1.1-6.6 mg/kg BW IM q6-24h (Kinsell, 1986)
Gp 0.2 mg/kg BW SC (Lumb and Jones, 1984)
H   0.5 mg/kg BW IM (Hofing, 1989)
M   5-10 mg/kg BW SC (Taber and Irwin, 1969)
    25-50 mg/kg BW IM (Dolowy et al, 1960)
N   3-6 mg/kg BW IM (USAF, 1976)
R   1-2 mg/kg BW IM (Clifford, 1984)
Rb 25 mg/kg BW IM (Produces myositis; CCAC, 1984)

Codeine

D   2.2 mg/kg BW SC (Jenkins, 1987)

M 20 mg/kg BW SC (Jenkins, 1987)
    60-90 mg/kg BW PO (Jenkins, 1987)
    20 mg/kg BW SC q4h (Flecknell, 1987)
R 25-60 mg/kg BW SC q4h (Jenkins, 1987)
    60-90 mg/kg BW SC q4h (Flecknell, 1991)

Diazepam

Bi 2-5 mg/kg BW IM (Cooper, 1984)
    1-1.5 mg/kg IV, IM (McDonald, 1989)
C 1 mg/kg BW IV to a maximum of 5 mg (Kinsell, 1986)
Ch 2.5 mg/kg BW IP (Green, 1982)
D 1 mg/kg BW IV to a maximum of 20 mg (Kinsell, 1986)
F 2 mg/kg BW IM (Flecknell, 1987; CCAC, 1984)
G 5 mg/kg BW IP (Flecknell, 1987; CCAC, 1984)
Go 0.5-1.5 mg/kg BW IM, IV (Swindle and Adams, 1988)
    15 mg/kg BW PO mixed in feed (NCSU, 1987)
Gp 5 mg/kg BW IP (Flecknell, 1987)
    2.5 mg/kg BW IP, IM (Green, 1982)
H 5 mg/kg BW IP (Flecknell, 1987; CCAC, 1984)
M 5 mg/kg BW IP (Green, 1979; Flecknell, 1987)
N 1 mg/kg BW IM (Flecknell, 1987)
    1 mg/kg BW IV (Green, 1982)
R 2 mg/kg BW IV (Flecknell, 1987)
    4 mg/kg BW IM, IP (Flecknell, 1987)
    2.5 mg/kg BW IM, IP (Weihe, 1987)
Rb 2 mg/kg BW IV (Flecknell, 1987)
    4 mg/kg BW IM, IP (Flecknell, 1987)
    5-10 mg/kg BW IM (Harkness and Wagner, 1983)
    5-10 mg/kg BW IM, IP (Green, 1982)
Rc 66-110 mg/kg BW PO (Balser, 1965)
Sh 0.5-1.5 mg/kg BW IM, IV (Swindle and Adams, 1988)
    15 mg/kg BW mixed with feed (NCSU, 1987)
Sw 0.5-10 mg/kg BW IM (Swindle and Adams, 1988)
    0.5-1.5 mg/kg BW IV (Swindle and Adams, 1988)

Diclofenac

Gp 2.1 mg/kg BW PO (Albengres et al, 1988)
M 8 mg/kg BW PO (Liles and Flecknell, 1992)
R 10 mg/kg BW PO (Liles and Flecknell, 1992)

Fenoprofen

D 0.5-1 mg/kg BW PO q24h (Jenkins, 1987)

Fentanyl

D 0.04-0.08 mg/kg BW SC, IM, IV q1-2h (Jenkins, 1987)
  0.001-0.003 mg/lb BW IM or slow IV (Kinsell, 1986)
N 0.05-0.10 mg/kg BW SC, IM (Jenkins, 1987)
Sw 0.02-0.05 mg/kg BW IM, IV (Swindle and Adams, 1988)

Fentanyl/droperidol (Innovar-Vet) (a preanesthetic dose of atropine may be necessary)

D 1 ml/7-10 kg BW IM (Kinsell, 1986)
  1 ml/12-30 kg BW IV (Kinsell, 1986)
F 0.15 ml/kg BW IM (Flecknell, 1987)
Gp 0.5-1.0 ml/kg BW IM (CCAC, 1984)
  0.08-0.66 ml/kg BW IM (Hughes, 1981)
  0.22 ml/kg BW IM (Sander, 1992)
H 0.01 ml/kg BW IP (CCAC, 1984) (CNS stimulation may occur; Hughes, 1981)
M 0.005 ml/kg BW IM (Jenkins, 1987)
  0.02-0.03 ml/g BW IM (Hughes, 1981)
N 0.1-0.2 ml/kg BW IM (CCAC, 1984)
  0.3 ml/kg BW IM (Flecknell, 1987)
R 0.13 ml/kg BW IM (Jenkins, 1987)
Rb 0.17 ml/kg BW IM (CCAC, 1984)
  0.15-0.17 ml/kg BW IM (Lewis and Jennings, 1972)
Sw 0.07 ml/kg BW IM (Swindle and Adams, 1988)

Fentanyl/fluanisone (Hypnorm)

F 0.5 ml/kg BW IM (Flecknell, 1987)
G 1 ml/kg BW IM, IP (Jenkins, 1987)
Gp 1 ml/kg BW IM (Jenkins, 1987; Flecknell, 1987)
H 1 ml/kg BW IM, IP (Jenkins, 1987)
M 0.01 ml/30g BW IP (Jenkins, 1987)
R 0.4 ml/kg BW IM, IP (Jenkins, 1987)
  0.2-0.5 ml/kg BW IM or 0.3-0.6 ml/kg BW IP (Flecknell, 1987)
Rb 0.5 ml/kg BW IM (Jenkins, 1987)

Flunixin

Bi 1-10 mg/kg IM. Can be repeated (Harrison and Harrison, 1986)

C   1 mg/kg BW PO, IV q24h (Haskins, 1987)
    0.3 mg/kg BW IM (Kinsell, 1986)
D   0.5-2.2 mg/kg BW IM, IV No repeat (Jenkins, 1987)
    1 mg/kg BW PO, IV q24h (Haskins, 1987)
M   2.5 mg/kg BW SC, IM try q12h (Flecknell, 1991)
N   0.5 mg/kg BW IM sid (Feeser and White, 1992)
    1 mg/kg BW IV bid (Fraser, 1991)
    Prosimians: 0.5 mg/kg BW IM sid (Feeser and White, 1992)
    10 mg/kg BW IM (Borchard et al, 1990)
R   1.1 mg/kg BW SC, IM q12h (Flecknell, 1991)
    2.5 mg/kg BW SC, IM (Liles and Flecknell, 1992)
Rb 1.1 mg/kg BW SC, IM try q 12h (Liles and Flecknell, 1992)

Hypnorm—*See* "fentanyl/fluanisone"

Ibuprofen

C   5 mg/kg BW PO q24h (Haskins, 1987)
D   10 mg/kg BW PO q24-48h (Jenkins, 1987)
    5 mg/kg BW PO q24h (Haskins, 1987)
Gp 10 mg/kg BW IM try q4h (Flecknell, 1991)
M   7.5 mg/kg BW PO (Jenkins, 1987)
    7.5 mg/kg BW PO try q4h (Flecknell, 1991)
    30 mg/kg BW PO (Liles and Flecknell, 1992)
R   10-30 mg/kg BW PO (Jenkins, 1987)
    10-30 mg/kg BW PO, try q4h (Flecknell, 1991)
Rb 10-20 mg/kg BW IV, try q4h (Flecknell, 1991)

Indomethacin

Gp 8.8 mg/kg BW PO (Albengres et al, 1988)
M   1 mg/kg BW PO (Liles and Flecknell, 1992)
R   2 mg/kg BW PO (Liles and Flecknell, 1992)
Rb 12.5 mg/kg BW PO (Keller et al, 1990)

Ketamine

Bi See under anesthetics.
C   10-30 mg/kg BW IM, IV (Kinsell, 1986)
Gp 25-30 mg/kg BW IM (Bauck, 1989)
    22-64 mg/kg BW IP (Sander, 1992)
H   60 mg/kg BW IM (Bauck, 1989)
N   5-40 mg/kg BW IM (Holmes, 1984)
Rb 30 mg/kg BW IM (Bauck, 1989)

Ketoprofen

Rb 1 mg/kg BW IM (Perrin et al, 1990)

Meclofenamic acid

C 2.2 mg/kg BW PO q24h (Haskins, 1987)
D 2.2 mg/kg BW PO q24h (Haskins, 1987)

> **Note:** Test dose-0.5 mg/lb sid for 5 days. If therapeutic results achieved, wait till signs exacerbate. Then drop dosage to 0.5 mg/lb qod till achieve signs of remission. Then drop to 0.5 mg/lb every third day for 1 week. If signs still remissed, drop dose to 0.5 mg/lb q4th day. If signs still remissed, drop dose to 0.5 mg/lb q5th day. When signs show exacerbation, back up one step and maintain that dose level (Kinsell, 1986)

Meperidine

C 2-10 mg/kg BW SC, IM q2h (Jenkins, 1987)
2-4 mg/kg BW IM, SC (Kinsell, 1986)
D 2-10 mg/kg BW SC, IM q2-3h (Jenkins, 1987)
6-10 mg/kg BW IM, SC (Kinsell, 1986)
Go 2-10 mg/kg BW SC, IM (Swindle and Adams, 1988)
Gp 20 mg/kg BW SC, IM q2-3h (Jenkins, 1987)
10-20 mg/kg BW SC, IM q2-3h (Flecknell, 1991)
H 20 mg/kg BW SC, IM q2-3h (Jenkins, 1987)
N 2-4 mg/kg BW IM q3-4h (Jenkins, 1987)
11 mg/kg BW IM (CCAC, 1984)
M 20 mg/kg BW SC, IM q2-3h (Jenkins, 1987)
10-20 mg/kg BW SC, IM q2-3h (Flecknell, 1991)
20-40 mg/kb BW IP (Clifford, 1984)
60 mg/kg BW IM (Hughs, 1981)
R 20 mg/kg BW SC, IM q2-3h (Jenkins, 1987)
10-20 mg/kg BW SC, IM q2-3h (Flecknell, 1991)
Rb 10 mg/kg BW SC, IM q2-3h (Jenkins, 1987)
10-20 mg/kg BW SC, IM q2-3h (Flecknell, 1991)
Sh 2-10 mg/kg BW SC, IM (Swindle and Adams, 1988)
Sw 4-10 mg/kg BW IM (Swindle and Adams, 1988)

Methadone

Gp 3-6 mg/kg BW SC (Jenkins, 1987)

H   3-6 mg/kg BW SC (Jenkins, 1987)

Midazolam

R   2 mg/kg BW IV (Flecknell, 1987)
        4 mg/kg BW IM, IP (Flecknell, 1987)
Rb 2 mg/kg BW IV (Flecknell, 1987)
        2 mg/kg BW intranasal (Robertson and Eberhart, 1994)
        4 mg/kg BW IM, IP (Flecknell, 1987)

Morphine

C   0.1 mg/kg BW SC, IM q4-6h (Jenkins, 1987; Flecknell, 1985)
        0.1 mg/kg BW IM, SC q6-7h; use with caution (Kinsell, 1986)
D   0.25-5.0 mg/kg BW IM, SC q4-6h (Jenkins, 1987; Flecknell,
        1985)
Gp   10 mg/kg BW SC, IM q2-4h (Jenkins, 1987; Flecknell, 1985)
        2-5 mg/kg BW SC, IM q4h (Flecknell, 1991)
H   10 mg/kg BW SC, IM q2-4h (Jenkins, 1987)
M   10 mg/kg BW SC q2-4h (Jenkins, 1987; Flecknell, 1985)
        2-5 mg/kg BW SC, hourly (Flecknell, 1991)
N   1-2 mg/kg BW SC q4h (Jenkins, 1987; Flecknell, 1985)
        3 mg/kg BW BW SC (Domino et al, 1969)
R   10 mg/kg BW SC q2-4h (Jenkins, 1987; Flecknell, 1985)
        2-5 mg/kg BW SC, hourly (Flecknell, 1991)
Rb 5 mg/kg BW SC, IM q2-4h (Jenkins, 1987; Flecknell, 1985)
        2-5 mg/kg BW SC, IM q2-4h (Flecknell, 1991)
Sw 0.2-0.9 mg/kg BW SC (Swindle and Adams, 1988)

Nalbuphine

D   0.5-2.0 mg/kg BW SC, IM, IV q3-8h (Jenkins, 1987)
M   4-8 mg/kg BW IM q4h (Flecknell, 1989)
R   2-5 mg/kg BW IM q4h (Flecknell, 1989)
        1-2 mg/kg BW IM q3h (Flecknell, 1991)
Rb 1-2 mg/kg BW IV q4-5h (Flecknell, 1989)
Sh   1 mg/kg SC q2-3h (Flecknell, 1989)

Naproxen

D   5 mg/kg BW loading dose, then 1.2-2.8 mg/kg BW PO q24h
        (Jenkins, 1987)

Gp   14.9 mg/kg BW PO (Albengres et al, 1988)
N   10 mg/kg BW PO q12h (Junge et al, 1992)
R   14.5 mg/kg BW PO (Borchard et al, 1990)

Oxymorphone

C   0.4-1.5 mg/kg BW SC, IM, IV (Jenkins, 1987)
D   0.22 mg/kg BW SC, IM, IV (Jenkins, 1987)
G   0.15 mg/kg BW IM (Trim et al, 1987)
H   0.15 mg/kg BW IM (Trim et al, 1987)
M   0.15 mg/kg BW IM (Trim et al, 1987)
N   Old World Monkeys: 0.15 mg/kg BW SC, IM, IV (Rosenberg, 1991)
   New World Monkeys: 0.075 mg/kg BW SC, IM, IV (Rosenberg, 1991)
R   0.15 mg/kg BW IM (Trim et al, 1987)
Sw   0.15 mg/kg BW IM (Swindle and Adams, 1988)

Pentazocine

C   2-3 mg/kg BW SC, IM, IV q4h (Jenkins, 1987)
   8 mg/kg BW IP q4h (Flecknell, 1985)
   1-3 mg/kg BW SC, IM, IV; IV duration 2-4 hrs (Kinsell, 1986)
D   2-3 mg/kg BW IM q4h (Jenkins, 1987; Flecknell, 1985)
   15 mg/kg BW PO q8h (Jenkins, 1987)
   1-3 mg/kg BW SC, IM, IV: IV duration 2-4 hrs (Kinsell, 1986)
M   10 mg/kg BW SC q3-4h (Jenkins, 1987; Flecknell, 1985)
   10 mg/kg BW SC, hourly (Flecknell, 1991)
N   2-5 mg/kg BW IM q4h (Jenkins, 1987; Flecknell, 1985)
R   10 mg/kg BW SC q4h (Jenkins, 1987; Flecknell, 1985)
   10 mg/kg BW SC, hourly (Flecknell, 1991)
Rb   10-20 mg/kg BW SC, IM q4h (Jenkins, 1987; Flecknell, 1985)
   5 mg/kg BW IV q2-4h (Flecknell, 1991)
Sw   2-5 mg/kg BW IM q4h (Swindle and Adams, 1988)

Pentobarbital sodium

C   2-4 mg/kg BW IV for sedation (Kinsell, 1986)
D   2-4 mg/kg BW IV for sedation (Kinsell, 1986)

Pethidine

Gp   20 mg/kg BW SC, IM q2-3h (Flecknell, 1987)

M   20 mg/kg BW SC, IM q2-3h (Flecknell, 1987)
N   2-4 mg/kg BW IM q3-4h (Flecknell, 1987)
R   20 mg/kg BW SC, IM q2-3h (Flecknell, 1987)
Rb 10 mg/kg BW SC, IM q2-3h (Flecknell, 1987)

Phenacetin
M   200 mg/kg BW PO q4h (Flecknell, 1987)
R   100 mg/kg BW PO q4h (Flecknell, 1987)

Phenylbutazone
C   15 mg/kg BW IV q8h (Haskins, 1987)
     10-14 mg/kg BW PO q12h (Kinsell, 1986)
D   15 mg/kg BW IV q8h (Haskins, 1987)
     22 mg/kg BW PO q8h (Haskins, 1987)
     6-7 mg/lb BW PO q8h with maximum dose of 800 mg per day,
       regardless of weight (Kinsell, 1986)
Gp 40 mg/kg BW PO (Wilhelmi, 1974)
M   30 mg/kg BW PO (Liles and Flecknell, 1992)
R   20 mg/kg BW PO (Liles and Flecknell, 1992)

Piroxicam
Gp 5.7 mg/kg BW PO (Albengres et al, 1988)
M   3 mg/kg BW PO (Liles and Flecknell, 1992)
R   3 mg/kg BW PO (Liles and Flecknell, 1992)

Telazol—*See* "tiletamine/zolazepam"

Tiletamine/zolazepam (Telazol)
Note: We recommend that users obtain the reference by Schobert, 1987, for the use of Telazol in 52 primate species, 21 cat species, 10 bear species, 8 dog species, 13 members of the Vierridae family, 9 reptile species, 10 species of the Bovidae family, 33 species of the Cervidae family, 36 bird species, and a table of various miscellaneous species. Not recommended in rabbits.

Tiletamine/zolazepam and xylazine (respectively)
H   20 mg/kg BW IP and 10 mg/kg BW IP (Forsythe et al, 1992)

Xylazine

Bi Used in combination with ketamine.

C 0.5 mg/lb BW IV (Kinsell, 1986)
1 mg/lb BW IM, SC (Kinsell, 1986)

D 0.5 mg/lb BW IV (Kinsell, 1986)
1 mg/lb BW IM, SC (Kinsell, 1986)

Go 0.05-1 mg/kg BW IM (Swindle and Adams, 1988); however, this
is considered unpredictable given IM
0.01 mg/kg BW IV (NCSU, 1987)

Gp 3-5 mg/kg BW IM (Harkness and Wagner, 1983)

H 4 mg/kg BW IM (Bauck, 1989)

M 4-8 mg/kg BW IM (Harkness and Wagner, 1983)
10 mg/kg BW IP (Flecknell, 1987)

N 1-2 mg/kg BW IM (Green, 1982; CCAC, 1984)

R 4-8 mg/kg BW IM (Harkness and Wagner, 1983)
1-3 mg/kg BW IM (Flecknell, 1987)

Rb 3-5 mg/kg BW IM (Harkness and Wagner, 1983)
5 mg/kg BW IM (Hughes, 1981)
1-3 mg/kg BW IM (Flecknell, 1987)

Sh 0.05-1 mg/kg BW IM (Swindle and Adams, 1988)
0.1-0.15 mg/kg BW slow IV (NCSU, 1987)

Sw 10 mg/kg BW IM (Swindle and Adams, 1988)

ANESTHETICS

Alphadolone/Alphaxalone—*See* "Saffan"

Avertin—*See* "tribromoethanol/amylene hydrate"

Azaperone and ketamine

M 75 mg/kg BW IM azaperone and 100 mg/kg BW IM ketamine (duration of anesthesia approx 1½ hrs) (Olson and Renchko, 1988)

R 50 mg/kg BW IM azaperone and 87 mg/kg BW IM ketamine. Give ¼ to 1½ times this dose depending on the length of anesthesia required (approx 1-6 hours) (Olson and Renchko, 1988)

Benzocaine

Am Larvae: 50 mg/l bath (dissolve in ethanol first) (Crawshaw, 1993)

Frogs, salamanders: 200-300 mg/l bath (Crawshaw, 1993)

Fi 20-50 ppm in water (Green, 1982)

Carbon dioxide

M Mix 1:1 CO_2:O_2 (Green, 1979)

Chloral hydrate

Am 1-2 mls of a 10% solution injected into dorsal lymph sac (Kaplan, 1969)

C 300 mg/kg BW IV (Borchard et al, 1990)

D   125 mg/kg BW IV (Borchard et al, 1990)
Go   50-300 mg/kg BW IV (Swindle and Adams, 1988)
Gp   200-300 mg/kg BW IP of 10% solution (Green, 1982)
H   270-360 mg/kg BW IP (Hughes, 1981)
M   400 mg/kg BW IP (Borchard et al, 1990)
R   200-300 mg/kg BW IP of 10% solution (Green, 1982)
Sh   50-300 mg/kg BW IV (Swindle and Adams, 1988)
Sw   100-300 mg/kg BW IV (Swindle and Adams, 1988)

Chloralose

C   75 mg/kg IV (Borchard et al, 1990)
D   80 mg/kg BW IV with 5 mg/kg BW IV thiopental sodium initially, then maintain anesthesia with additional chloralose (1 ml/sec IV); respirator required at this dose of chloralose (Grad et al, 1988)
Go   45-62 mg/kg BW IV (Swindle and Adams, 1988)
M   114 mg/kg BW IP (Hughes, 1981)
R   55 mg/kg BW IP (Borchard et al, 1990)
Rb   80-100 mg/kg BW IV of 1% solution (Green, 1982)
Sh   45-62 mg/kg BW IV (Swindle and Adams, 1988)
Sw   55-86 mg/kg BW IV (Swindle and Adams, 1988)

Ethyl alcohol

Am   Frogs and toads: Immerse in 10% solution (Kaplan, 1969)

Etomidate

M   30 mg/kg BW IP (Green et al, 1981)

Etorphine (M-99)

Re   Turtles: 0.5-5.0 mg total dose (for approx. 1.8 kg animal) (Marcus, 1981)
Snakes: 2-15 mg total dose IPP (Marcus, 1981)

Fentanyl/droperidol (Innovar-Vet)

Ch   0.20 ml/kg BW IM (Green, 1982)
F   0.5 ml/kg BW IM (Green, 1982)

Gp 0.66-0.88 ml/kg BW IM (Hughes, 1981)
     0.5-1.0 ml/kg BW IM (CCAC, 1984)
H Not recommended (Thayer et al, 1972)
M 0.05 ml/g BW IM (Hughes, 1981)
N 1.0 ml/9 kg BW IM (Melby and Altman, 1976)
R 0.02-0.06 ml/100 g BW IP (Wixson et al, 1987)
     0.3 ml/kg BW IM (Hughes, 1981)
Rb 0.10-0.50 ml/kg BW IM (Green, 1982)
Sw 0.10 ml/kg BW IM (Swindle and Adams, 1988)

Fentanyl/droperidol and diazepam

H 1 ml/kg BW IP fentanyl/droperidol and 5 mg/kg BW IP diazepam
     (Green, 1982)

Fentanyl/fluanisone (Hypnorm)

Gp 0.5 ml/kg BW IM

     Note: Addition of 1-2 mg/kg BW IP or IM diazepam is advisable
     (Cooper, 1984)

M 0.5 ml/kg BW IM

     Note: Addition of 1-2 mg/kg BW IP or IM diazepam is advisable
     (Cooper, 1984)

R 0.5 ml/kg BW IM (Cooper, 1984)

Fentanyl and metomidate

M 60 and 0.002-0.006 mg/kg BW SC, respectively (Green et al, 1981)

Halothane

Am Terrestrial species: 4-5% in anesthetic chamber to effect (Craw-
     shaw, 1993)

Hexobarbital

Am 120 mg/kg BW intravascularly (Kaplan, 1969)

M 100 mg/kg BW IP (Taber and Irwin, 1969)
R 100 mg/kg BW IP (Ben et al, 1969)

Hypnorm—*See* "fentanyl/fluanisone"

Inactin
R 80 mg/kg BW IP (Flecknell, 1987)
100-110 mg/kg BW IP (Ellison et al, 1987)

Isoflurane
Am Terrestrial species: 4-5% in anesthetic chamber to effect (Crawshaw, 1993)
Bi 1.5-2.5% (to effect). Inhalant drug of choice (Nemetz, 1990)

Ketamine (Used alone in mammals, we have found that ketamine is not usually adequate for deep anesthesia, Eds.)
Am 50-150 mg/kg SC, IM (Crawshaw, 1993)
Bi 10-50 mg/kg BW IM (Fowler, 1978; Cooper, 1984)
0.03-0.04 mg/g BW IM for light anesthesia (Nemetz, 1990)
0.07-0.10 mg/g BW IM for surgical anesthesia in birds <100 g BW (Nemetz, 1990)
0.05-0.08 mg/g BW IM for surgical anesthesia in birds 200-500 g BW (Nemetz,1990)
0.03-0.06 mg/g BW IM for surgical anesthesia in birds >500 g BW (Nemetz, 1990)

Note: An excitatory phase may occur during recovery.

F 20-30 mg/kg BW IM (Green, 1982)
20-30 mg/kg BW IM for immobilization (Flecknell, 1987)
20-35 mg/kg BW IM (Andrews and Illman, 1987)
G 200 mg/kg BW IM for immobilization (Flecknell, 1987)
Go 22-44 mg/kg BW IM (Swindle and Adams, 1988)
Gp 44 mg/kg BW IM, atropine recommended (Weisbroth and Fudens, 1972)
100-200 mg/kg BW IM for immobilization (Flecknell, 1987)
H 10-30 mg/100 g BW IP (Strittmatter, 1972)
200 mg/kg BW IP for immobilization (Flecknell, 1987)

M 44 mg/kg BW IM for sedation (Weisbroth and Fudens, 1972)
   100-200 mg/kg BW IP (Hughes, 1981)
   200 mg/kg BW IM for immobilization (Flecknell, 1987)
   50 mg/kg BW IV (Hughes, 1981)

N 10-30 mg/kg BW IM (Welshman, 1985)
   African green (*Cercopithecus* spp.): 25-30 mg/kg BW IM (Cramlet and Jones, 1976)
   Baboon (*Papio* spp.): 7.5-10 mg/kg BW IM (Cramlet and Jones, 1976)
   Chimpanzee (*Pan troglotydes*): 10-15 mg/kg BW IM (Cramlet and Jones, 1976)
   Cynomolgus macaque (*Macaca fascicularis*): 20-25 mg/kg BW IM (Cramlet and Jones, 1976)
   Gorilla (*Gorilla gorilla*): 12-15 mg/kg BW IM (Cramlet and Jones, 1976)
   Patas (*Erythrocebus patas*): 5-7.5 mg/kg BW IM (Cramlet and Jones, 1976)
   Rhesus macaque (*Macaca mulatta*): 20-25 mg/kg BW IM (Cramlet and Jones, 1976)
   Squirrel monkey (*Saimiri sciureus*): 25-30 mg/kg BW IM (Cramlet and Jones, 1976)

R 44 mg/kg BW IM (Weisbroth and Fudens, 1972)
   100 mg/kg BW IM for immobilization (Flecknell, 1987)
   75 mg/kg BW IP (Waterman and Livingston, 1978)

Rb 44 mg/kg BW IM (Weisbroth and Fudens, 1972)
   50 mg/kg BW IM for immobilization (Flecknell, 1987)
   25 mg/kg BW intranasal for light surgical anesthesia (Robertson and Eberhart, 1994)

Rc 5-27 mg/kg BW IM (use higher doses for longer anesthetic duration) (Evans and Evans, 1986)

Re Snakes: 88-110 mg/kg BW IM (for 3.6-4.5 kg animals) (Marcus, 1981)
   Snakes: 22-44 mg/kg BW IM (for < 0.9 kg animals) (Marcus, 1981)
   50-130 mg/kg BW IM (Page, 1993)
   Tortoises and turtles: 15-60 mg/kg BW IM (Fowler, 1978)
   Tortoises: 20-80 mg/kg BW IM (Page and Mautino, 1990)
   Chelonians: 20-60 mg/kg BW IM (Page, 1993)

Sh 22-44 mg/kg BW IM (Swindle and Adams, 1988)

Sw 15-25 mg/kg BW IM (Swindle and Adams, 1988)
   15-20 mg/kg BW IV (Swindle and Adams, 1988)

Ketamine and acepromazine (respectively)

G 75 mg/kg BW IM and 3 mg/kg BW IM (Flecknell, 1987)
Gp 125 mg/kg BW IM and 5 mg/kg BW IM (Flecknell, 1987)
H 150 mg/kg BW IM and 5 mg/kg BW IM (Flecknell, 1987)
M 100 mg/kg BW IM and 2.5 mg/kg BW IM (Flecknell, 1987)
N *Varecia* and *Propithecus* (not *Lemur*)—4 mg/kg BW IM and 0.4
     mg/kg BW IM (Feeser and White, 1992)
R 75 mg/kg BW IM and 2.5 mg/kg BW IM (Flecknell, 1987)
     30 mg/kg BW IM and 3 mg/kg BW IM (Roman and Osborn, 1987)
Rb 75 mg/kg BW IM and 5 mg/kg BW IM (Flecknell, 1987)
Rc 8-10 mg/kg BW IM and 2.2 mg/kg BW IM (Evans and Evans, 1986)

Ketamine and azaperone—*See* "azaperone and ketamine"

Ketamine and detomidine (respectively)

R 60 mg/kg BW IM and 10 mg/kg BW IM in males (Cox et al, 1994)
    40 mg/kg BW IM and 5 mg/kg BW IM in females (Cox et al, 1994)

Ketamine and diazepam (respectively) (Use two syringes: not miscible)

Bi Use anesthetic dose and 1-1.5 mg/kg BW IM to improve muscle
     relaxation (Nemetz, 1990)
Ch 20 mg/kg BW IM, IP and 5 mg/kg BW IM, IP (Flecknell, 1987)
F 25 mg/kg BW IM and 2 mg/kg BW IM (Flecknell, 1987)
G 50 mg/kg BW IM and 5 mg/kg BW IP (Flecknell, 1987)
Gp 100 mg/kg BW IM and 5 mg/kg BW IM (Flecknell, 1987)
M 200 mg/kg BW IM and 5 mg/kg BW IP (Flecknell, 1987)
N 15 mg/kg BW IM and 1 mg/kg BW IM (Flecknell, 1987)
R 40-80 mg/kg BW IP and 5-10 mg/kg BW IP (Wixson et al, 1987)
Rb 25 mg/kg BW IM and 5 mg/kg BW IM (Flecknell, 1987)

Ketamine, tiletamine/lorazepam, and xylazine (respectively)

Sw 2.2 mg/kg BW IM, 4.4 mg/kg BW IM, and 2.2 mg/kg BW IM (Ko
     et al, 1993)

Ketamine and xylazine (respectively)

Bi 0.05 mg/g BW IM and 0.01 mg/g BW IM. Use less volume in birds
>500 g BW (Nemetz, 1990)
40 mg/kg BW IM and 10 mg/kg BW IM (Heaton and Brauth, 1991)

F 25 mg/kg BW IM; 2 mg/kg BW IM (Moreland and Glaser, 1985)

G 50 mg/kg BW IM and 2 mg/kg BW IM (Flecknell, 1987)

Gp 40 mg/kg BW IM and 5 mg/kg BW SC (Flecknell, 1987)
50 mg/kg BW IP and 5 mg/kg BW IP (Strother and Stokes, 1989)

H 200 mg/kg BW IP and 10 mg/kg BW IP (Flecknell, 1987)

M 200 mg/kg BW IM and 10 mg/kg BW IP (Flecknell, 1987)

Note: High mortality possible

90-120 mg/kg BW IM and 10 mg/kg BW IM (Harkness and
Wagner, 1989)

R 40-80 mg/kg BW IP and 5-10 mg/kg BW IP (Wixson et al, 1987)
90 mg/kg BW IM and 10 mg/kg BW IM (Flecknell, 1987)

Rb 50 mg/kg BW IM and 10 mg/kg BW IM (Lipman et al, 1987)
10 mg/kg BW IV and 3 mg/kg BW IV (Flecknell, 1987)
10 mg/kg BW intranasal and 3 mg/kg BW intranasal (Robertson and
Eberhart, 1994)

Rc 5-8 mg/kg BW IM and 1.5-3 mg/kg BW IM (Evans and Evans,
1986)
5.5 mg/kg BW IM and 5.5 mg/kg BW IM (Evans and Evans, 1986)

Ketamine, xylazine, and acepromazine

M 30 mg/kg BW IM ketamine, 6 mg/kg BW IM xylazine, and 1 mg/kg
BW IM acepromazine (O'Rourke et al, 1994)

Rb 35 mg/kg BW IM ketamine, 5 mg/kg BW IM xylazine and 0.75
mg/kg BW IM acepromazine (Marini et al, 1989)

Note: This provides approximately 30% longer anesthesia and recovery than ketamine and xylazine alone.

M-99—*See* "etorphine"

Medetomidine and propofol (respectively)

Rb 0.25 mg/kg BW IM and 4 mg/kg BW IV (Ko et al, 1992)

Medetomidine, midazolam, and propofol (respectively)

Rb 0.25 mg/kg BW IM, 0.5 mg/kg BW IM, and 2 mg/kg BW IV (Ko et al, 1992)

Methohexital

Gp 31 mg/kg BW IP (Flecknell, 1987)
M 6 mg/kg BW IV (Flecknell, 1987)
N 10 mg/kg BW IV (Flecknell, 1987)
R 7-10 mg/kg BW IV (Flecknell, 1987)
Rb 10 mg/kg BW IV (Flecknell, 1987)

Methoxyflurane

C ~3% for induction: 0.5% by inhalation for maintenance (Kinsell, 1986)
D 3% for induction: 0.5% by inhalation for maintenance (Kinsell, 1986)
M To effect (Williams, 1976)
R To effect (Williams, 1976)

Metomidate

M 30-50 mg/kg BW IP (Green et al, 1981)

Pentobarbital sodium

Am Frogs and toads: 60 mg/kg in dorsal lymph sac (Marcus, 1981; Kaplan, 1969)
Bo 12-28 mg/kg BW IV (Schultz, 1989)
C 30 mg/kg IV to effect for anesthesia (Kinsell, 1986)
D 30 mg/kg IV to effect for anesthesia (Kinsell, 1986)
F 36 mg/kg BW IP (Andrews and Illman, 1987)
 30 mg/kg BW IV (Green, 1982)
G 6 mg/100 g BW IP up to 6 mg maximum (Norris, 1987)
Go 25-30 mg/kg BW IV (Swindle and Adams, 1988)
Gp 28 mg/kg BW IP (Croft, 1964)
H 9 mg/100 g BW IP, boost with 1.2 mg/100 g BW (Whitney, 1963)
M 40-85 mg/kg BW IP (Cunliffe-Beamer, 1983)
 50 mg/kg BW IP followed by a dose of 25 mg/kg BW SC for longer procedures (45-50 min) (Taber and Irwin, 1969)
 Neonates (1-4 days): 5 mg/kg BW IP (Taber and Irwin, 1969)

N   5-15 mg/kg BW IV (Flecknell, 1987)
R   30-40 mg/kg BW IP (Wixson et al, 1987)
Rb 28 mg/kg BW IV, IP (Croft, 1964)
Rc 30 mg/kg BW IP (Evans and Evans, 1986)
Re Turtles: 16 mg/kg BW IC, IP (Marcus, 1981)
      Snakes: 15-30 mg/kg BW IPP (Marcus, 1981)
Sh 25-30 mg/kg BW IV (Swindle and Adams, 1988)
      15-30 mg/kg BW IV, lower dose for castrated animals (NCSU, 1987)
Sw 25-35 mg/kg BW PO (Swindle and Adams, 1988)
      30 mg/kg BW IP (Swindle and Adams, 1988)
      20-30 mg/kg BW IV (Swindle and Adams, 1988)

Pentobarbital and chlorpromazine

M   40-60 mg/kg BW IP and 25-50 mg/kg IM (Harkness and Wagner, 1989)

Propofol

Rb 7.5-15 mg/kg BW IV (Adam et al, 1990)
      1.5 mg/kg BW IV bolus followed by 0.2-0.6 mg/kg/min continuous infusion (Blake et al, 1988)

Saffan (alphadolone/alphaxalone)

Bi 8.0 mg/kg BW IV; incremental doses up to 25 mg/kg BW maximum (Cooper, 1984)
C   9 mg/kg BW IV initially, followed by multiple 3 mg/kg BW IV doses as needed to maintain anesthesia (from product information)
      18 mg/kg BW IM initially, followed by multiple 3 mg/kg BW IV doses as needed to maintain anesthesia (from product information)
Ch 20-30 mg/kg BW IM (Green, 1982)
D   Not suitable for use in dogs (Glaxovet guide to Saffan)
F   12-15 mg/kg BW IM initially, followed by multiple 6-8 mg/kg BW IV doses as needed to maintain anesthesia (Green, 1982)
G   80-120 mg/kg BW IP (Flecknell, 1987)
Gp 10-20 mg/kg BW IV (Green, 1982)
      40 mg/kg BW IP (Flecknell, 1987)
H   150 mg/kg BW IP (Flecknell, 1987)

M 5 mg/kg BW IV (with incremental doses up to 20 mg/kg maximum (Cooper, 1984)

90 mg/kg BW IP (Green, 1982)

N 6-9 mg/kg BW IV initially, followed by supplemental doses to effect as needed to maintain anesthesia (from product information)

12-18 mg/kg BW IM initially, followed by multiple 6-9 mg/kg BW IV doses as needed to maintain anesthesia (from product information)

R 5 mg/kg BW IV (with incremental doses up to 20 mg/kg max (Cooper, 1984); has been given by slow IV drip for periods up to 10 hours without tolerance or cumulation developing (Green, 1982)

Rb 6-9 mg/kg BW IV (Green, 1982); High mortality possible (Flecknell, 1987)

Re 9.0 mg/kg BW IV (Frye, 1981)

12-18 mg/kg BW IM (Cooper, 1984)

Chelonians: 9-18 mg/kg BW IM (Page, 1993)

Lizards: 9-18 mg/kg BW IM (Page, 1993)

Telazol—*See* "tiletamine/zolazepam"

Thiamylal

N 25 mg/kg BW IV (Hughes et al, 1975)

Thiopental

D 6-12 mg/lb BW IV; lower dose with preanesthetic tranquilization (Kinsell, 1986)

Go 20-25 mg/kg BW IV (Swindle and Adams, 1988)

M 25-50 mg/kg BW IV (Taber and Irwin, 1969)

25 mg/kg BW IV (Hughes, 1981)

50 mg/kg BW IP (Williams, 1976)

N 15-20 mg/kg BW IV (Flecknell, 1987)

22-25 mg/kg BW (Hatch, 1966)

R 30 mg/kg BW IV (Flecknell, 1987)

Rb 28 mg/kg BW IV, IP (Croft, 1964)

Re Snakes: 15-25 mg/kg BW IPP (Marcus, 1981)

Sh 20-25 mg/kg BW IV (Swindle and Adams, 1988)

Sw 24-30 mg/kg BW IP (Swindle and Adams, 1988)

5-19 mg/kg BW IV (Swindle and Adams, 1988)

Tiletamine

Rc   10-12 mg/kg BW IM (Evans and Evans, 1986)

Tiletamine/zolazepam (Telazol)

Note: We recommend that users obtain the reference by Schobert, 1987, for the use of Telazol in 52 primate species, 21 cat species, 10 bear species, 8 dog species, 13 members of the Vierridae family, 9 reptile species, 10 species of the Bovidae family, 33 species of the Cervidae family, 36 bird species, and a table of various miscellaneous species.

F   22 mg/kg BW IM (Payton and Pick, 1989)
G   60 mg/kg BW IM (Hrapkiewicz et al, 1989)
Gp   10-30 mg/kg IM (Fowler, 1978)
H   Not recommended (Silverman et al, 1983)
M   Not recommended (Silverman et al, 1983)
N   2-6 mg/kg BW IM (Ialeggio, 1989)
R   20-40 mg/kg BW IP (Silverman et al, 1983)
Rb   Not generally recommended (except intranasal); nephrotoxicity
         (Doerning et al, 1990, 1992)
         10-25 mg/kg BW IM (Fowler, 1978)
         10 mg/kg BW intranasal (no renal compromise) (Robertson and
         Eberhart, 1994)
Re   Chelonians: 10-20 mg/kg BW IM (Page, 1993)
         Snakes: 22 mg/kg BW IM (Marcus, 1981)
         Snakes: 10-20 mg/kg BW IM (Page, 1993)
         Lizards: 30 mg/kg BW IM (Page, 1993)
Sh   2.2 mg/kg BW IM (Schultz, 1989)
Sw   6.6-11 mg/kg BW IM following xylazine 2 mg/kg BW IM (Schultz,
         1989)

Tiletamine/zolazepam and xylazine

H   30 mg/kg BW IP and 10 mg/kg BW IP (Forsythe et al, 1992)
Rb   15 mg/kg BW IM and 5 mg/kg BW IM (Popilskis et al, 1991)
Sw   4.4 mg/kg BW IM and 2.2 mg/kg BW IM (Ko et al, 1993)

Tribromoethanol

G   250-300 mg/kg BW IP (1.25% solution) (Flecknell, 1987)
M   125 mg/kg BW IP (0.25% solution) (Flecknell, 1987)
         250 mg/kg BW IP (Taber and Irwin, 1969)
         0.2 ml/10 g BW IP of a 1.2% solution (Papaioannou and Fox, 1993)

R 300 mg/kg BW IP (Flecknell, 1987)

Tribromoethanol/amylene hydrate (Avertin)

Note: No longer available commercially but can be made. For concentrated solution (66 2/3%) dissolve 1 g 2,2,2-tribromoethanol in 0.5 g amylene hydrate. Take 0.5 ml concentrate and mix with 39.5 ml sterile saline (this is now a 1.25% solution). If solution falls below pH 5, discard. Warning: Stored solutions are known to be unstable and potentially hepatotoxic. Frequent use may induce chemical peritonitis.

G 250-300 mg/kg BW IP of 1.25% solution (Flecknell, 1987)
M 0.2 ml/10g BW IPof 1.25% solution (The Jackson Laboratory)
R 300 mg/kg BW IP (Flecknell, 1987)

Tricaine methanesulphonate (MS 222)

Am Immerse in 0.1% solution (Kaplan, 1969)
   50-150 mg/kg BW SC, IM (Crawshaw, 1993)
   Tadpoles, newts: 200-500 mg/l bath to effect (Crawshaw, 1993)
   Frogs, salamanders: 500-2000 mg/l bath (buffer with NaHCO₃) (Crawshaw, 1993)
   Toads: 1-3 g/l bath (buffer with NaHCO₃) (Crawshaw, 1993)
Fi Immerse in 25-100 mg/L water (Klontz, 1964)
Re Snakes: 200-300 mg/kg BW IPP (Marcus, 1981)

Urethane

Am Frogs and toads: Immerse in 1-2% solution (Kaplan, 1969)
   Frogs and toads: Inject 0.04-0.12 ml/g BW of 5% solution into dorsal lymph sac (Kaplan, 1969)
F 1500 mg/kg BW IP for acute use only (Andrews and Illman, 1987)
Fi Immerse in 5-40 mg/L water (Klontz, 1964)
Gp 1500 mg/kg BW IV, IP (Flecknell, 1987)
R 1000 mg/kg BW IP (Flecknell, 1987)
Rb 1000 mg/kg BW IV, IP (Flecknell, 1987)
Re Turtles: 2.8 g/kg PO (Marcus, 1981)
   2.4 g/kg IV (Marcus, 1981)
   1.7 g/kg IC (Marcus, 1981)
   2.8 g/kg IP (Marcus, 1981)

ANTI-INFECTIVES

Acyclovir

Bi 80 mg/kg BW PO tid by gavage for 7-14 days (Nemetz, 1990)

20 mg/kg IV tid (Nemetz, 1990)

Amikacin

Bi 40 mg/kg BW IM sid or bid (Burke, 1986); for psittacines use lower dose listed below (Nemetz, 1990)

22 mg/kg BW q12h (Schultz, 1989)

15-20 mg/kg BW IM bid (Nemetz, 1990)

N 2.3 mg/kg BW IM sid (Wissman and Parsons, 1992)

Re Snake: 5 mg/kg BW IM loading dose followed by 2.5 mg/kg BW IM q72h for 5 treatments (Bennett, 1989)

Tortoises: 5 mg/kg BW IM q48h for 7-14 days (Page and Mautino, 1990)

Amoxicillin

Bi 150 mg/kg BW PO bid for 7-14 days (Nemetz, 1990)

Bo 10 mg/kg BW PO q8-12h (Schultz, 1989)

3-5 mg/lb BW IM, SC sid (Kinsell, 1986)

400 mg/100 lb BW PO bid (Sundlof et al, 1991)

62.5 mg (contents of one prepackaged syringe) into each affected quarter q12h for a maximum of three treatments (Sundlof et al, 1991)

C 5-10 mg/lb BW PO q12h (Kinsell, 1986)

5 mg/lb BW IM, SC sid (Kinsell, 1986)

D 5 mg/lb BW PO q12h (Kinsell, 1986)

5 mg/lb BW SC, IM sid (Kinsell, 1986)

Gp Toxic (Flecknell, 1987)
H Toxic (Flecknell, 1987)
M 100 mg/kg BW SC, IM bid (Flecknell, 1987)
N 7 mg/kg BW SC (Flecknell, 1987)
   10 mg/kg BW PO (Flecknell, 1987)
   11 mg/kg BW PO bid (Fraser, 1991)
   11 mg/kg BW SC, IM sid (Fraser, 1991)
R 150 mg/kg BW SC, IM bid (Flecknell, 1987)

Amphotericin B

Bi 1.5 mg/kg BW IV sid, bid (tid for raptors) for 3-7 days; SC sid
   advocated by some for 3-4 weeks; 1 mg/ml in saline to nebulize
   15 min bid (Nemetz, 1990)
   1.0 mg/kg BW IT sid for up to 30 days (Nemetz, 1990)

   Note: Dilute drug in sterile water at 1 mg/ml (Nemetz, 1990)

C 0.25-0.5 mg/kg BW 2-3 times/week on alternate days, slow IV, IP
   with 5% dextrose and water (Kinsell, 1986)
D 0.25-0.5 mg/kg BW 2-3 times/week on alternate days, slow IV, IP
   with 5% dextrose and water (Kinsell, 1986)
   0.25-1.0 mg/kg BW IV sid (Johnson et al, 1981)
N 0.25-1.0 mg/kg BW IV sid (Johnson et al, 1981)

Ampicillin

Bi Ampicillin sodium—100 mg/kg BW IM, IV q4h (Nemetz, 1990;
   Burke, 1986)
   250 mg/8 oz drinking water (change daily)(Burke, 1986)
   150-200 mg/kg BW PO bid, tid (Nemetz, 1990)
Bo Ampicillin trihydrate—5-10 mg/lb BW IM q8h for up to 7 days
   (Kinsell, 1986)
C Ampicillin sodium—3 mg/lb BW IV, IM q8-12h (Kinsell, 1986)
   Ampicillin trihydrate—3-8 mg/lb BW IM, SC q8-12h or 10-30
   mg/lb BW PO q8-12h (Kinsell, 1986)
D Ampicillin sodium—3 mg/lb BW IV, IM q8-12h (Kinsell, 1986)
   Ampicillin trihydrate—3-8 mg/lb BW IM, SC q8-12h or 5-10 mg/lb
   BW PO q6-8h (Kinsell, 1986)
F 5 mg/kg BW SC sid (McKellar, 1989)
Gp May cause enterocolitis (Bartlett et al, 1978)
   6 mg/kg BW SC tid for 5 days (Young et al, 1987)
H Toxic (Flecknell, 1987)

M   2-10 mg/100 g BW PO bid (Russell et al, 1981)
      50-150 mg/kg BW SC bid (Flecknell, 1987)
N   30 mg/kg BW IM sid for 5 days (Welshman, 1985)
      5 mg/kg BW IM bid (Flecknell, 1987)
      20 mg/kg BW IM, IV, PO tid (Johnson et al, 1981)
R   50-150 mg/kg BW SC bid (Flecknell, 1987)
      50 mg/adult rat IP sid for 10 days (Rettig et al, 1989)
Rb 22-44 mg/kg BW PO in divided doses (Bowman and Lang, 1987)
      10-25 mg/kg BW IM sid for 5-7 days (Bowman and Lang, 1987)
Re 3-6 mg/kg BW IM, SC sid until 48 h beyond recovery (Marcus, 1981)
      20 mg/kg BW IC bid for 7-9 days (Snipes,1984)
      Tortoises: 20 mg/kg BW IM sid for 7-14 days (Page and Mautino, 1990)

Amprolium

Bi 4 ml/gal water of 9.6% solution for 5 days (Nemetz, 1990)
Bo 10 mg/kg BW daily in feed for 5 days (Schultz, 1989)
D   100-200 mg/kg BW per day PO in food or water for 7-10 days (Kinsell, 1986)

Apramycin

Bi 1 g/gal water for 7-10 days in turkeys (Nemetz, 1990)
      12.5 mg/4 oz water for 7-10 days in small birds (Nemetz, 1990)
      12.5 mg/8 oz water for 7-10 days in large birds (Nemetz, 1990)
Sw 150 g/ton of food. Use for 14 days (Sundlof et al, 1991)

Carbenicillin

Bi 200 mg/kg BW PO bid (Burke, 1986)
      100 mg/kg BW IM bid, tid (Nemetz, 1990)
      100-200 mg/kg BW PO bid (tablet, bitter taste) (Nemetz, 1990)
D   10-15 mg/lb BW PO q8h or 5-10 mg/lb BW IV q8h (Kinsell, 1986)
Re 100 mg/kg BW initially, then 75 mg/kg IM sid or IV bid (Frye, 1981)
      Tortoises: 200-400 mg/kg BW IM q48h for 7-14 days (Page and Mautino, 1990)

Carnidazole

Bi 10 mg single dose per pigeon, for trichomoniasis (Nemetz, 1990)

Cefazolin

Bi   50 mg/kg BW IM tid (Nemetz, 1990)
Gp   100 mg/kg BW IM bid (Fritz et al, 1987)
N   25 mg/kg BW IM, IV bid for 7-10 days (Univ of Washington, 1987)

Cefotaxime

Bi   100 mg/kg BW IM bid (Nemetz, 1990)
N   100-200 mg/kg BW IM tid-qid (Pernikoff and Orkin, 1991)
Re   Tortoises: 20-40 mg/kg BW IM sid for 7-14 days (Page and Mautino, 1990)

Ceftazidime

N   *Propithecus:* 50 mg/kg BW IM, IV tid (Feeser and White, 1992)
    50 mg/kg BW IM tid (Feeser and White, 1992)

Ceftizoxime

N   75-100 mg/kg BW IM bid for 7 days (Univ of Washington, 1987)

Cephalexin

Bi   50 mg/kg BW PO qid (Burke, 1986)
    35-50 mg/kg BW PO qid (Nemetz, 1990)
C   35 mg/kg BW PO q12h (Kinsell, 1986)
D   35 mg/kg BW PO q12h (Kinsell, 1986)
Gp   50 mg/kg BW IM sid for 14 days (Richardson, 1992)
M   60 mg/kg BW PO bid (Flecknell, 1987)
N   20 mg/kg BW PO bid (Flecknell, 1987)
R   60 mg/kg BW PO bid (Flecknell, 1987)
Rb   15-20 mg/kg BW PO bid (Flecknell, 1987)

Cephaloridine

F   15 mg/kg BW IM sid (McKellar, 1989)
G   30 mg/kg BW IM bid (Flecknell, 1987)
Gp   10-25 mg/kg BW IM sid for 5-7 days (Harkness and Wagner, 1977)
    15-25 mg/kg BW SC sid (Bauck, 1989)
    12.5 mg/kg BW IM sid for 14 days (Dixon, 1986)
H   May cause enterocolitis (Bartlett et al, 1978)
    10 mg/kg BW IM bid (Holmes, 1984)
    30 mg/kg BW IM bid (Flecknell, 1987)

M 30 mg/kg BW IM bid (Flecknell, 1987)
N 11 mg/kg BW IM bid (Melby and Altman, 1976)
  20 mg/kg BW IM bid (Flecknell, 1987)
R 30 mg/kg BW IM bid (Flecknell, 1987)
Rb 10-25 mg/kg BW IM, SC sid for 5 days (Bowman and Lang, 1987)
Re 10 mg/kg BW IM, SC bid (Frye, 1981)

Cephalothin

Bi 100 mg/kg BW IM qid (Burke, 1986)
  100 mg/kg BW IM tid, qid (Nemetz, 1990)
C 40-80 mg/kg BW/day IM, IV q8-12h (Kinsell, 1986)
D 40-80 mg/kg BW/day IM, IV q8-12h (Kinsell, 1986)
Rb 13 mg/kg BW IM qid for 6 days (Bowman and Lang, 1987)
Re 20-40 mg/kg BW IM bid (Frye, 1981)

Chloramphenicol palmitate (not for use in food animals)

Bi 75-100 mg/kg BW PO bid, tid, qid (Nemetz, 1990)
C 15-20 mg/lb BW PO q8-12h (Kinsell, 1986)
D 20-25 mg/lb BW PO q6-8h (Kinsell, 1986)
F 40 mg/kg BW PO tid for 14 days (Krueger et al, 1989)
  50 mg/kg BW PO bid for 10 days (Krueger et al, 1989)
G 50 mg/kg BW PO bid (Bauck, 1989)
Gp 50 mg/kg BW PO bid (Bauck, 1989)
  50 mg/kg BW PO tid (Russell et al, 1981)
H 20 mg/100 g BW PO tid (Russell et al, 1981)
  50 mg/kg BW PO bid (Bauck, 1989)
M 20 mg/100 g BW PO tid (oral suspension)(Russell et al, 1981)
  100 mg/200 ml drinking water for 3-5 days (Williams, 1976)
  50 mg/kg BW PO bid (Bauck, 1989)
N 50 mg/kg BW PO bid (Flecknell, 1987)
R 20 mg/100 g BW PO tid (Russell et al, 1981)
  50 mg/kg BW PO bid (Bauck, 1989)
Rb 50 mg/kg BW PO sid for 5-7 d (Harkness and Wagner, 1983)
  50 mg/kg BW PO bid (Bauck, 1989)
Re Tortoises: 20 mg/kg BW PO bid for 7 to 14 days (Page and Mautino, 1990)

Chloramphenicol succinate (not for use in food animals)

Bi 80 mg/kg BW IM bid or tid (Burke, 1986)
  50 mg/kg BW IV tid (Nemetz, 1990)

C 10 mg/kg BW IM, IV q12h (Kinsell, 1986)
D 10 mg/kg BW IM, IV q12h (Kinsell, 1986)
Fi 75 mg/kg BW PO sid in feed for 14 days (CCAC, 1984)
G 30 mg/kg BW IM bid (Flecknell, 1987)
    50 mg/60 ml drinking water for two weeks (Williams, 1976)
    50 mg/kg BW SC bid (Bauck, 1989)
Gp 20 mg/kg BW IM bid (Flecknell, 1987)
    50 mg/kg BW SC bid (Bauck, 1989)
H 30 mg/kg BM IM bid (Flecknell, 1987)
    50 mg/kg BW SC bid (Bauck, 1989)
M 50 mg/kg BW IM bid (Flecknell, 1987)
    50 mg/kg BW SC bid (Bauck, 1989)
N 25 mg/kg BW IV bid for 10 days (DaRif and Rush, 1983)
    50 mg/kg BW IM bid for 10 days (DaRif and Rush, 1983)
    30 mg/kg BW IM tid (Welsh, 1985)
    110 mg/kg BW IM qid for 5-10 days for pneumococcal memin-
      goencephalitis (Ialeggio, 1989)
R 50 mg/kg BW IM bid (Flecknell, 1987)
    50 mg/kg BW SC bid (Bauck, 1989)
Rb 30 mg/kg BW IM sid for 5-7 d (Harkness and Wagner, 1983)
    50 mg/kg BW SC bid (Bauck, 1989)
    50 mg/kg BW SC, IM, IV tid (Russell et al, 1981)
Re Toads: 5 mg/100 g BW initially, then 3 mg/100 g BW PO bid for 5
    days (Marcus, 1981)
    Turtles: 40 mg/kg BW IM, IP bid for 7 days (Marcus, 1981)
    Tortoises: 20 mg/kg BW IM bid for 7-14 days (Page and Mautino,
    1990)

Chlorhexidine

Bi 15-20 ml of 2% solution/gal water. Flock antifungal treatment for
    2-4 weeks (Nemetz, 1990)

Chlortetracycline

B 1 mg/ml active drug in drinking water Raphael, 1981)
    10 g/ton feed (Flatt et al, 1974)
Bi 5,000 ppm in food for 30-45 days (Burke, 1986)
    250 mg/pint water as sole source. Must be mixed fresh bid or tid
    (Nemetz, 1990)
    100 g/20 lb mash (Nemetz, 1990)
R 50 mg/100 ml drinking water as prophylaxis (Hawk, 1991)

Ciprofloxacin

Bi 20-40 mg/kg BW PO bid (Nemetz, 1990)
N 16-20 mg/kg BW PO q12h in sterile water (Kelly et al, 1992)
Rb 50 mg/kg BW IM tid for 4 days (Strunk et al, 1985)
40 mg/kg BW IM tid for 28 days (Norden et al, 1985)
40 mg/kg BW IM bid for 17 days (Bayer et al, 1985)

Clindamycin

Bi 100 mg/kg BW PO sid, bid (Nemetz, 1990)
Gp May cause enterotoxic cecitis (Bartlett, 1979)

Dimetridazole

H 500 mg/L drinking water (La Regina et al, 1980)
Rb 0.025% solution prepared using 45 g active ingredient/50 gal drinking water (Williams, 1979)

Doxycycline

Bi 18-26 mg/kg BW oral syrup PO bid in psittacines (Burke, 1986)
25 mg/kg BW oral syrup PO bid or 50 mg/kg BW oral syrup PO sid (Nemetz, 1990)
22-44 mg/kg BW IV sid or bid (Burke, 1986)
22-44 mg/kg BW IV once, then switch to oral dose (Nemetz, 1990)
N 5 mg/kg BW PO divided bid day 1; 2.5 mg/kg BW the following days (Wolff, 1990)

Enrofloxacin

Bi 15-20 mg/kg BW PO bid (Nemetz, 1990)
2.5-5 mg/kg BW IM bid (Rosskopf, 1989)
GP 5-10 mg/kg BW PO (Dorrestein, 1992)
100 mg/l in water (Dorrestein, 1992)
H 5-10 mg/kg BW PO (Dorrestein, 1992)
100 mg/l in water (Dorrestein, 1992)
M 85 mg/kg BW SC bid for 14 days (Goelz et al, 1994)
85 mg/kg/d PO in deionized water for 14 days (Goelz et al, 1994)
N 5 mg/kg BW IM, PO q24h for 5 days (Line, 1993)
5 mg/kg BW by gastric intubation sid for 10 days (Line et al, 1992)

Rb 10 mg/kg BW bid (Mladinich, 1989)
5 mg/kg BW PO bid (Broome et al, 1991)
5-10 mg/kg BW PO (Dorrestein, 1992)
100 mg/l in water (Dorrestein, 1992)

Erythromycin

Bi 200 mg/10 ml saline for nebulization tid (15 min) (Nemetz, 1990)

Note: Do not inject IM; severe muscle necrosis.

40-80 mg/kg BW PO bid (Nemetz, 1990)
C 5-10 mg/lb BW PO q8h (Kinsell, 1986)
D 5-10 mg/lb BW PO q8h (Kinsell, 1986)
Fi 100 mg/kg BW in feed for 21 days (CCAC, 1984)
Gp May cause enterocolitis (Bartlett et al, 1978)
H May cause enterocolitis (Bartlett et al, 1978)
N 40 mg/kg BW IM sid (Welshman, 1985)
75 mg/kg BW PO bid for 10 days (Univ of Washington, 1987)

Ethambutol

Bi 15 mg/kg BW PO for up to one year (Rosskopf, 1989)
N 22.5 mg/kg BW PO sid in grape juice (reduce dose by ⅓ after 6 weeks) (Wolf et al, 1988)

Flucytosine

Bi Psittacines: 100-250 mg/kg BW PO (hidden in yogurt) bid for 14 days (Nemetz, 1990)
Raptors: 18-30 mg/kg BW PO qid for 14 days (Nemetz, 1990)

Furazolidone

Bi 20 mg/400 g BW PO sid (Nemetz, 1990)
N 10-15 mg/kg BW PO sid (Melby and Altman, 1976)
Rb 2.5 g/100 lb feed
400 mg/pt in drinking water
Re 25-40 mg/kg BW PO sid (Frye, 1981)

Gentamicin

Bi   **Note:** No longer recommended for parenteral use in pet birds. May be used for sinus flushes or nebulization (10 mg/kg IT sid with 1 ml/10 ml saline) (Nemetz, 1990)

Most large: 5 mg/kg BW IM bid or tid (Burke, 1986)
Most small: 10 mg/kg BW IM bid or tid (Burke, 1986)
Raptors: 2.5 mg/kg BW IM tid (Burke, 1986)
40 mg/kg BW PO sid or bid (Burke, 1986)
25 mg/4 oz water for 7-10 days (Nemetz, 1990)

C   2 mg/lb BW IM, SC q12h the first day, then sid (Kinsell, 1986)
D   2 mg/lb BW IM, SC q12h the first day, then sid (Kinsell, 1986)
G   0.5 mg/100 g BW IM sid (Russell et al, 1981)
5-8 mg/kg BW SC sid (Bauck, 1989)
Gp 5-8 mg/kg BW SC sid (Bauck, 1989)
H   May cause enterocolitis (Bartlett et al, 1978)
0.5 mg/100 g BW IM sid (Russell et al, 1981)
5-8 mg/kg BW SC sid (Bauck, 1989)
M   0.5 mg/100 g BW IM sid (Russell et al, 1981)
1.2 g/l drinking water for 3 days (Russell et al, 1981)
5-8 mg/kg BW SC sid (Bauck, 1989)
N   2 mg/kg BW IM, IV bid for 10 days (DaRif and Rush, 1983)
2 mg/kg BW IM tid for 7-10 days (Ialeggio, 1989)
Baboon: 3 mg/kg BW IM bid (Ralph et al, 1989)
R   0.5 mg/100 g BW IM sid (Russell et al, 1981)
5-8 mg/kg BW SC sid (Bauck, 1989)
Rb 4 mg/kg BW IM sid (Russell et al, 1981)
5-8 mg/kg BW SC sid (Bauck, 1989)
Re Nonchelonian: 2.5 mg/kg BW q72h supplemented with parenteral fluids (Frye, 1981; Bennett, 1989)
Chelonians: 10 mg/kg q48h supplemented with parenteral fluids (Frye, 1981)
Chelonians: 10-20 mg/15 ml normal saline bid nebulized for 30 min (Snipes, 1984)
Tortoises: 5 mg/kg BW IM q72h for 7 to 14 days (Page and Mautino, 1990)

Griseofulvin

C   20 mg/kg BW/day PO sid for 6 weeks, or 140 mg/kg/week once each week for 6 weeks. See note below. (Kinsell, 1986)
D   20 mg/kg BW/day PO sid for 6 weeks, or 140 mg/kg/week once each week for 6 weeks. See note below. (Kinsell, 1986)

Note: For D and C, qualified individuals have found that the above doses may not be adequate and suggest the dosage of 65 mg/kg/day. One should consider treatment for at least 6 weeks duration. The once-a-week treatment is to be discouraged. (Kinsell, 1986) One should also consider immune deficiency diseases if treatment appears ineffective (Eds.).

F   25 mg/kg BW PO (Ryland and Gorham, 1978)

Gp 75 mg/kg BW PO sid for 2 wk (Harkness and Wagner, 1983)
        1.5% in DMSO applied topically bid for 14 days (Post and Saunders, 1979)

M   25 mg/100 g BW PO q10d (Russell et al, 1981)

N   20 mg/kg BW PO sid (Johnson et al, 1981)
        200 mg/kg BW PO once every 10 days (Johnson et al, 1981)

R   25 mg/100 g BW PO q10d (Russell et al, 1981)

Rb 25 mg/100 g BW PO q10d (Russell et al, 1981)
        2.5 mg/100 g BW PO for 14 days (Russell et al, 1981)

Isoniazid

N   5 mg/kg BW PO in divided doses (Johnson et al, 1981)
        Chimpanzees: 15-25 mg/kg BW PO bid (Fineg, 1966)
        25 mg/kg BW PO sid in grape juice (reduce dose by ⅓ after 6 weeks) (Wolf et al, 1988)

Kanamycin

Bi 10-20 mg/kg BW IM bid (Burke, 1986)
        10-50 mg/L drinking water (change daily) for 3-5 days (Burke, 1986)

C   2.5 mg/lb BW SC q12h (Kinsell, 1986)

D   2.5 mg/lb BW SC q12h (Kinsell, 1986)

N   7.5 mg/kg BW IM bid (Johnson et al, 1981)

Re 10-15 mg/kg/day in divided doses IV, IM, IP (Frye, 1981)

Ketoconazole

Bi 50 mg/kg BW PO sid (Nemetz, 1990)
        25-30 mg/kg BW PO bid (Nemetz, 1990)

C   10-20 mg/kg BW PO q8-12h (Kinsell, 1986)

D   10-20 mg/kg BW PO q8-12h (Kinsell, 1986)

Re Tortoises: 30 mg/kg BW PO sid for 2 to 4 weeks (Page and Mautino, 1990)

Lincomycin

Bi Raptors: 100 mg/kg BW PO sid (Burke, 1986)
100 mg/kg BW PO bid for 7-10 days (Nemetz, 1990)

C 10 mg/lb BW PO q12h or 7 mg/lb BW PO q8h (Kinsell, 1986)
10 mg/kg BW IM q12h (Kinsell, 1986)
5-10 mg/lb BW slow IV in 5% glucose or normal saline (Kinsell, 1986)

Note: Do not continue therapy longer than 12 days. May cause pseudomembranous colitis.

D 10 mg/lb BW PO q12h or 7 mg/lb BW PO q8h (Kinsell, 1986)
10 mg/kg BW IM q12h (Kinsell, 1986)
5-10 mg/lb BW slow IV in 5% glucose or normal saline (Kinsell, 1986)

Note: Do not continue therapy longer than 12 days. May cause pseudomembranous colitis.

N 5-10 mg/kg BW IM bid (Williams, 1976)
Re 6 mg/kg BW IM bid, sid (Frye, 1981)

Methicillin

N 50 mg/kg BW IM bid for 7 days (Univ of Washington, 1992)

Metronidazole

Bi Lovebirds: 10 mg/kg BW IM sid for 3 days (Nemetz, 1990)
Cockatiels: 35-50 mg/kg BW IM sid for 5 days; repeat in 2-4 weeks (Nemetz, 1990)

D 60 mg/kg BW PO sid for 5 days (Kinsell, 1986)
F 35 mg/kg BW PO sid for 5 days (Bell, 1994)
Gp 20 mg/kg BW PO, SC sid (Richardson, 1992)
M 2.5 mg/ml drinking water for 5 days (Roach et al, 1988)
N 35-50 mg/kg/day BW PO bid for 10 days (Holmes, 1984)
Re 125-275 mg/kg BW PO once, may be repeated at 7-10 day intervals for 1-2 more treatments (Frye, 1981)
Tortoises: 250 mg/kg BW PO once, repeat in 2 weeks (Page and Mautino, 1990)

Minocycline

N 4 mg/kg BW PO (Whitney et al, 1977)

  15 mg/kg BW PO q12h for 7 days (Junge et al, 1992)

Rb 6 mg/kg BW IV q8h (Nicolau et al, 1993)

Neomycin

Bi 10 mg/kg BW PO bid or tid (Burke, 1986)

  1-8 drops Biosol/oz water for 1-3 days (Nemetz, 1990)

C 5-7 mg/lb BW PO q6-24h (Kinsell, 1986)

D 5-7 mg/lb BW PO q6-24h (Kinsell, 1986)

F 10-20 mg/kg BW PO (Ryland and Gorham, 1978)

G 100 mg/kg BW PO sid (Flecknell, 1987)

  10 g/gal drinking water for 5 days, then 5 g/gal for an additional 5 days (Russell et al, 1981)

Gp 5 mg/300-400 g animal PO bid for 5 days (Farrar and Kent, 1965)

  10 mg/kg BW PO sid (Flecknell, 1987; McKellar, 1989)

  30 mg/kg SC (Flecknell, 1987)

  5 mg/kg BW PO bid (Richardson, 1992)

H 5 ml Biosol/100 ml drinking water for 5 days, then give half dose for 5 more days (Russell et al, 1981)

  125 mg/L in drinking water (La Regina et al, 1980)

  10 mg in 0.25 ml water/40 g animal sid via intragastric admin. (Sheffield and Beveridge, 1962)

  10 mg in 0.5 g cheese pellet/40 g animal sid for 5 wk for prophylaxis

  10 mg/kg BW PO sid (Flecknell, 1987)

M 2 mg/ml in drinking water for 14 days; prepare fresh daily (Barthold, 1980)

  10 g/gal drinking water for 5 days, then 5 g/gal for an additional 5 days (Russell et al, 1981)

  50 mg/kg BW SC sid (McKellar, 1989)

N 10 mg/kg BW PO bid (Flecknell, 1987)

R 50 mg/kg BW IM bid (Flecknell, 1987)

  10 g/gal drinking water for 5 days, then 5 g/gal for an additional 5 days (Russell et al, 1981)

Nitrofurantoin

C 1-2 mg/lb BW PO q8h with food (Kinsell, 1986)

D 1-2 mg/lb BW PO q8h with food (Kinsell, 1986)

Gp 50 mg/kg BW sid for 3 days (Richardson, 1992)

N 2-4 mg/kg BW IM, IV tid (Johnson et al, 1981)
R 0.2% in feed for 6-8 weeks (Russell et al, 1981)

Nitrofurazone

Bi ⅛ to ¼ tsp of 9.3% soluble powder/L of water (change daily; Burke, 1986)
2 tsp of 4.59% soluble powder/gal water for 7-14 days; use 50% of this dose for lories and mynahs (Nemetz, 1990)
N 11 mg/kg BW PO sid (Melby and Altman, 1976)
Rb 11 mg/kg BW PO sid (Melby and Altman, 1976)

Norfloxacin

M 200 mg/kg BW IM bid (our interpretation of Fromtling et al, 1985)

Nystatin

Bi 100,000 IU/500 g BW PO bid for 7-14 days (Nemetz, 1990)
100,000 IU/300 g BW PO tid for 7-14 days (Nemetz, 1990)
N 200,000 units PO qid until 2 days following recovery (Fraser, 1991)

Oxytetracycline

Bi 200 mg/kg BW IM sid (one dose)(Burke, 1986)
50-100 mg/kg BW SC every 3 days; slough will occur within 21 days (Nemetz, 1990)
200 mg/kg BW PO bid to qid (Nemetz, 1990)
Bo 7-11 mg/kg BW/day not to exceed 4 consecutive days (Schultz, 1989)
G 800 mg/L drinking water (Williams, 1976)
20 mg/kg BW SC sid (McKellar, 1989)
Gp 5 mg/kg BW IM bid (Merck Veterinary Manual, 1979)
H 20 mg/kg BW SC sid (McKellar, 1989)
M 400 mg/L drinking water given continuously (Williams, 1976)
100 mg/kg BW SC bid (Flecknell, 1987)
N 10 mg/kg BW SC, IM (Flecknell, 1987)
R 60 mg/kg BW SC q72h of long acting drug (Liquimycin LA-200) (Curl et al, 1988)
Rb 30-100 mg/kg BW in divided doses PO (Bowman and Lang, 1987)
400-1000 mg/L drinking water (Bowman and Lang, 1987)
15 mg/kg BW SC, IM (Flecknell, 1987)

Re   6-10 mg/kg BW IV, IM sid (Frye, 1981)

Sh   7-11 mg/kg BW/day not to exceed 4 consecutive days (Schultz, 1989)

Penicillin

Bi   Penicillin G, Procaine—TOXIC in caged birds (Nemetz, 1990)

Bo   Penicillin G, Procaine—20,000-40,000 u/kg BW IM q12h (Schultz, 1989)

Penicillin G, Procaine and Penicillin G, Benzathine 20,000-40,000 u/kg BW SC q48h (Schultz, 1989)

C   Penicillin G, Procaine—40,000 u/kg BW IM q24h (Kinsell, 1986)

D   Penicillin G, Potassium—20,000 u/kg BW IM, IV (drip) q4-6h (Kinsell, 1986)

Penicillin G, Procaine—40,000 u/kg BW IM sid (Kinsell, 1986)

Penicillin G, Procaine and Penicillin G, Benzathine—1 ml/10-25 lbs BW IM, SC repeat in 48 hours (Kinsell, 1986)

Gp   May cause enterotoxic cecitis (Bartlett, 1979)

M   Penicillin, Potassium—100,000 IU/kg BW IM bid (do not use procaine penicillin) (Russell et al, 1981)

Penicillin, Potassium—60,000 u/mouse IM (Taber and Irwin, 1969)

N   Penicillin G, Procaine—20,000 u/kg BW IM bid (Johnson et al, 1981)

Penicillin G, Benzathine—40,000 u/kg BW IM every 3 days (Johnson et al, 1981)

R   Penicillin, Potassium—100,000 IU/kg BW IM bid (Russell et al, 1981)

15,000 IU oral penicillin/20 ml drinking water (Williams, 1976)

Rb   Penicillin G, Procaine and Penicillin G, Benzathine—42,000 or 84,000 IU/kg BW SC once each week for 3 weeks (Cunliffe-Beamer and Fox, 1981)

Penicillin G, Procaine and Penicillin G, Benzathine—"FloCillin"-2 ml per 10 lbs BW IM, SC every other day (Russell et al, 1981)

Penicillin G, Procaine—60,000 u/kg BW IM sid for 10 days (Jaslow et al, 1981; Welch et al, 1987)

Penicillin G, Procaine—50,000 IU/kg BW sid (Bauck, 1989)

Re   Penicillin G, Procaine and Penicillin G, Benzathine—10,000 u total penicillin activity/kg BW IM at 24-72 h intervals (Frye, 1981)

Penicillin G, Potassium—10,000-20,000 u/kg BW IM, SC tid or qid (Frye, 1981)

Sh   Penicillin G, Procaine and Penicillin G, Benzathine—10,000 or 20,000 u/kg BW IM q3 or 6d respectively (Schultz, 1989)

Sw Penicillin G, Procaine and Penicillin G, Benzathine—10,000-40,000 u/kg BW IM q3d (Schultz, 1989)

Piperacillin

Bi 100 mg/kg BW IM bid (Nemetz, 1990)
N 100-150 mg/kg BW IM, IV bid for 7-10 days (Univ of Washington, 1987)
  80-100 mg/kg BW IM, IV tid for 7-10 days (Univ of Washington, 1987)

Polymyxin B

Bi Budgies: 115 IU IM sid for 6 days (Nemetz, 1990)
  Budgies: 500,000 IU in 10 ml saline and 2.5 ml mucomyst for nebulization (Nemetz, 1990)
Rb 3 mg/300-400 g animal PO bid for 5 days (Farrar and Kent, 1965)

Rifampin

Bi 10-20 mg/kg BW PO bid (Rosskopf, 1989)
N 22.5 mg/kg BW PO sid in grape juice (reduce by 1/3 after six weeks) (Wolf et al, 1988)

Spectinomycin

Bi 2 g/gal water sid (Nemetz, 1990)
  1 mg/10 g BW IM sid for 5-10 days (Nemetz, 1990)
D 2.5-5 mg/lb BW IM q12h (Kinsell, 1986)

Streptomycin sulfate

Bi 10-15 mg/kg BW IM bid (Burke, 1986)

  30 mg/kg BW IM bid. Use in poultry only (Nemetz, 1990)
  10-20 mg/kg BW IM bid for 7 days (Rosskopf, 1989)
Fi 30-40 mg/kg BW IP sid (CCAC, 1984)
M 4-5 mg/adult mouse SC sid (McDougall et al, 1967)
Rb 10 mg/kg BW IM every 4 hours (CCAC, 1984)
Re 10 mg/kg BW IM bid (Frye, 1981)

Succinylsulfathiazole

Gp 0.1% in drinking water (Williams, 1976)

Sulfachlorpyridazine

Bi 0.25 tsp/l water for 5-10 days (Scultz, 1989)
      0.75 tsp/quart water for 5-10 days (Nemetz, 1990)

Sulfadiazine and pyrimethamine

M 100-200 mg/100 g feed and 30 mg/100 g feed respectively (Hawk, 1991)

Mi Toxic

R 100-200 mg/100 g feed and 30 mg/100 g feed respectively (Hawk, 1991)

Sulfadimethoxine

Bi 20 mg/kg BW PO bid (Burke, 1986)
     1 mg/30 g BW PO bid (Nemetz, 1990)

C 25 mg/lb BW IM, IP, PO, SC the first day, then 12.5 mg/lb BW q24h for 6 days (Kinsell, 1986)

D 25 mg/lb BW IM, IP, PO, SC the first day, then 12.5 mg/lb BW q24h for 6 days (Kinsell, 1986)

F 300 mg/kg BW daily in drinking water for two weeks (Bell, 1994)

Mi Toxic

Rb 75-100 mg/kg BW PO sid for 7 days (Rossof, 1974)

Re 90 mg/kg BW IV, IM sid first day, then 45 mg/kg BW sid days 2-6 (Frye, 1981)

Sulfamerazine

Fi 240 mg/kg BW sid in feed for 14 days (CCAC, 1984)

Gp 40 ml 12.5% solution/gal drinking water (Russell et al, 1981)

M 0.02% in drinking water (Flecknell, 1987)

Mi Toxic

R 0.02% in drinking water (Flecknell, 1987)

Sulfamethazine

Bi 30 mg/oz solution PO full strength instead of drinking water for 5-7 days (Burke, 1986)

C 50 mg/kg BW PO, IV q12h of 12.5% solution (Kinsell, 1986)

D 50 mg/kg BW PO, IV q12h of 12.5% solution (Kinsell, 1986)

Gp 12.5%—Add 4 ml/ 500 ml drinking water for 1-2 weeks (Williams, 1976)

   12.5%—Add 1.33-4.14 ml/L drinking water (Melby and Altman, 1976)

   166-517 mg/L drinking water (CCAC, 1984)

H 665-800 mg/L drinking water (CCAC, 1984)

M 12.5%—Dilute 1 ml with 49 ml water and give 0.5 ml diluted solution to 30 g mouse bid (Russell et al, 1981)

   12.5%—Add 5 ml/pt in drinking water (100 mg/kg BW PO) (Russell et al, 1981)

   450-1200 mg/L drinking water (CCAC, 1984)

Mi Toxic

N 66 mg/kg BW PO bid (CCAC, 1984)

R 12.5%—Add 5 ml/pt in drinking water (100 mg/kg BW PO) (Russell et al, 1981)

   665-950 mg/L drinking water (CCAC, 1984)

Rb 12.5%—Add 5 ml/pt in drinking water (100 mg/kg BW PO) (Russell et al, 1981)

   900-1350 mg/L drinking water (CCAC, 1984)

Re 0.5 g/kg BW PO sid first day, the 0.25 g/kg BW second through fourth day (Frye, 1981)

Sulfaquinoxaline

Bi Poultry: 0.0125%-0.025% in drinking water (Schultz, 1989)

Bo 10 g/100 lbs BW PO daily for 3-5 days (Schultz, 1989)

Gp 0.25-1.0 g/L drinking water for 30 days (Schuckman, 1977)

Mi Toxic

Rb 0.05% in drinking water (Patton, 1979)

   6 mg/lb BW PO for 5-7 days (Russell et al, 1981)

Re 0.04% in drinking water for 3-5 days (Frye, 1981)

Sh 10 g/100 lbs BW PO daily for 3-5 days (Schultz, 1989)

Sw 0.0125%-0.025% in drinking water (Schultz, 1989)

Sulfasalazine

N 30 mg/kg BW PO bid (Isaza et al, 1992)

Sulfisoxazole

N 50 mg/kg BW PO sid (Johnson et al, 1981)

Tetracycline

Am 1 mg/6 g BW PO (stomach tube) bid for 7 days (mix in small volume of distilled water) (Marcus, 1981)

Bi 250 mg/kg BW of oral suspension bid (Burke, 1986)

   1 tsp powder/gal water for 5-10 days; mixed fresh bid to tid (Nemetz, 1990)

C 10-25 mg/lb BW PO q8-12h (Kinsell, 1986)

D 10-25 mg/lb BW PO q8-12h (Kinsell, 1986)

G 250 mg/100 ml drinking water for 14 days (Williams, 1976)

   2 mg/100 g BW PO or IM (Clifford, 1973)

   20 mg/kg BW PO bid (Bauck, 1989)

Gp 112-350 mg/L drinking water (CCAC, 1984)

   20 mg/kg BW PO bid (Bauck, 1989)

   50 mg/kg BW PO by dropper divided into three doses (Richardson, 1992)

   5 mg/kg BW IM bid (Richardson, 1992)

H 400 mg/L in drinking water (La Regina et al, 1980)

   20 mg/kg BW PO bid (Bauck, 1989)

M 3-5 mg/ml in drinking water for 5-7 days (Harkness and Wagner, 1983)

   1 mg/ml in drinking water for 7 days (Barthold, 1980)

   20 mg/kg BW PO bid (Bauck, 1989)

   100 mg/kg BW SC sid (McKellar, 1989)

N 20-25 mg/kg BW PO bid-tid for 7-10 days (Johnson et al, 1981; Univ of Washington, 1987)

   25 mg/kg BW IM, IV bid (Univ of Washington, 1987)

R 450-643 mg/L drinking water (CCAC, 1984)

   20 mg/kg BW PO bid (Bauck, 1989)

   100 mg/kg BW SC (McKellar, 1989)

Rb 30-100 mg/kg BW in divided doses PO (Bowman and Lang, 1987)

   20 mg/kg BW PO bid (Bauck, 1989)

   500-900 mg tetracycline powder in dextrose/L drinking water. Fresh twice daily and protect from light. (Bauck, 1989)

Re 25-50 mg/kg BW PO bid until 48 h past recovery (Marcus, 1981)

Ticarcillin

Bi 200 mg/kg BW IM, IV bid to qid (Burke, 1986)

Tobramycin

Bi 10 mg/kg BW IM bid (Nemetz, 1990)

Gp 30 mg/kg BW q24h (Kapusnik et al, 1988)

Trimethoprim
N 75 mg/kg IM sid (Welsh, 1985)

Trimethoprim and sulfadiazine
C 5 mg/lb BW sid (Kinsell, 1986)
D 30 mg/kg BW/day PO; in severe infections use one-half daily dose q12h; adm. 2-3 days after signs subside but not more than 14 consecutive days (Kinsell, 1986)
1 ml/5 lbs BW of oral suspension (Kinsell, 1986)
1 ml/20 lbs SC sid of 24% injectable (Kinsell, 1986)
F 30 mg/kg BW PO or oral suspension (Bell, 1994)
G 30 mg/kg BW SC sid (Bauck, 1989)
Gp 0.5 ml/kg BW SC of 240 mg/ml solution (Flecknell, 1987)
30 mg/kg BW SC sid (Bauck, 1989)
H 30 mg/kg BW SC sid (Bauck, 1989)
M 0.5 ml/kg BW SC of 240 mg/ml solution (Flecknell, 1987)
N 0.2 ml/kg BW SC of 240 mg/ml solution (Flecknell, 1987)
0.1 ml/kg BW SC of 240 mg/ml solution for 7-10 days (Ialeggio, 1989)
Prosimians—25 mg/kg BW SC, IM sid (Feeser and White, 1992)
R 0.5 ml/kg BW SC of 240 mg/ml solution (Flecknell, 1987)
Rb 0.2 ml/kg BW SC bid of 240 mg/ml solution (Flecknell, 1987)
30 mg/kg BW SC sid (Bauck, 1989)
Re Tortoises: 30 mg/kg BW IM, PO q48h for 7 to 14 days (Page and Mautino, 1990)

Trimethoprim and sulfamethoxazole (dosed on sulfa concentration)
Bi 100 mg/kg BW PO bid (Burke, 1986)
80 mg/kg BW PO bid, tid (Nemetz, 1990)
44 mg/kg BW IM sid, bid (Nemetz, 1990)
G 15 mg/kg BW PO bid (Bauck, 1989)
Gp 15 mg/kg BW PO bid (Bauck, 1989)
H 15 mg/kg BW PO bid (Bauck, 1989)
Rb 15 mg/kg BW PO bid (Bauck, 1989)
N *Lemur* and *Varecia:* 50 mg/kg BW PO sid (Feeser and White, 1992)

Re   Tortoises: 30 mg/kg BW IM, PO q48h for 7-14 days (Page and
Mautino, 1990)

Tylosin

Bi   10-40 mg/kg BW IM bid or tid (Burke, 1986)

Bo   17.6 mg/kg BW/day IM not to exceed 5 days (Schultz, 1989)

C   1-5 mg/lb BW IM q12-24h (Do not mix with any other solution)
(Kinsell, 1986)
10-20 mg/lb BW/day PO divided q6-8h (Kinsell, 1986)

D   1-5 mg/lb BW IM q12-24h (Do not mix with any other solution)
(Kinsell, 1986)
10-20 mg/lb BW/day PO divided q6-8h (Kinsell, 1986)

G   10 mg/100 g BW PO for 21 days (Russell et al, 1981)
10 mg/kg BW IM, SC sid (McKellar, 1989)

H   100 mg/kg BW PO sid (Flecknell, 1987)
10 mg/100 g BW PO for 21 days (Russell et al, 1981)
10 mg/kg BW IM, SC sid (McKellar, 1989)

M   0.2-0.8 mg/100 g BW IM bid (Russell et al, 1981)
10 mg/kg BW SC bid (Flecknell, 1987)
10 mg/100 g BW PO for 21 days (Russell et al, 1981)

N   10 mg/kg BW IM bid (Welshman, 1985)

R   5 g/L in drinking water mixed with dextrose, give 100 mls treated
water to each rat daily (Carter et al, 1986)
10 mg/kg BW SC bid (Flecknell, 1987)
10 mg/100 g BW PO for 21 days (Russell et al, 1981)

Re   25 mg/kg BW IM, PO sid for 7 days (Marcus, 1981)

Sw   8.8 mg/kg BW IM q12h not to exceed 3 days (Schultz, 1989)

Vancomycin

H   20 mg/kg BW PO by gavage (Boss et al, 1994)

Rb   50 mg/kg BW IV q8h (Nicolau et al, 1993)

PARASITICIDES

Albendazole
N   25 mg/kg BW PO for 5 days (Wolff, 1990)

Amprolium
Bi   9.6% Solution—4 ml/gal water for 5 days (Nemetz, 1990)

   Note: Supplement with B vitamins

Bo   5 mg/kg BW daily in feed for 21 days prophylaxis (Schultz, 1989)
       10 mg/kg BW daily in feed for 5 days for treatment (Schultz, 1989)
D   100-200 mg/kg BW PO sid in food or water for 7-10 days (Kinsell, 1986)
F   19 mg/kg BW daily PO sid or in drinking water (Bell, 1994)
Rb   9.6% Solution—1 ml/15 lb BW PO for 5 days (Williams, 1979)

Bunamidine
C   25-50 mg/kg BW PO, single dose given on an empty stomach (after 3-4 h fast) (Kinsell, 1986)
D   25-50 mg/kg BW PO, single dose given on an empty stomach (after 3-4 h fast) (Kinsell, 1986)
M   1000 ppm in the diet for 18 days (Hawk, 1991)
N   25 mg/kg BW PO (Williams, 1976)
Re   25-50 mg/kg BW PO, not more often than once every 2-3 weeks (Frye, 1981)

Captan

Gp 1:200 dilution of 20% aqueous solution as a dip once each month for 4 months (Hawk, 1991)

R 1:200 dilution of 20% aqueous solution as a dip once each month for 4 months (Hawk, 1991)

Carbaryl

Bi Lightly dust body, wings, and legs. Add 1 tsp-2 tbs to nest box (Nemetz, 1990)

M Dust with 5% powder or dilute 1:1 with talc (Harknes and Wagner, 1983)

R Dust with 5% powder or dilute 1:1 with talc (Harkness and Wagner, 1983)

Rb Dust with 5% powder or dilute 1:1 with talc (Harkness and Wagner, 1983)

Clorsulon (8.5% orall drench)

Bi 20 mg/kg BW PO given once, repeat in 14 and 28 days (Clipshaw, 1989)

Crotamiton

Bi Topical application for scaly face mites every 3rd day to affected areas for 2 weeks, then once weekly for 5 weeks (avoid feathered areas) (Nemetz, 1990)

Note: Ivermectin is the drug of choice.

Decoquinate

F 0.5 mg/kg BW daily mixed in moist food (Bell, 1994)

Diazinon

M 0.03% as a spray or dip (Hawk, 1991)

R 0.03% as a spray or dip (Hawk, 1991)

Dichlorvos —*Also see* Vapona pest strip (DDVP)

C 5 mg/lb BW PO (Kinsell, 1986)

D   12-15 mg/lb BW PO in adults (Kinsell, 1986)
     5 mg/lb BW PO in puppies (Kinsell, 1986)

M   500 mg/kg food for 24 hours, repeat in 12 and 24 days (Wagner, 1970)

N   10-15 mg/kg BW PO for 2-3 days (Russell et al, 1981)
     30 mg/kg BW PO once (Melby and Altman, 1976)

R   0.5 mg/g food for 1 day (Wagner, 1970)

Rc 30 mg/kg BW PO (Evans and Evans, 1986)

Re 12.5 mg/kg BW PO daily for 2 doses (Frye, 1981)

Diethylcarbamazine

C   25-50 mg/lb BW PO once, repeat in 10-20 days for ascarids (Kinsell, 1986)

D   3-5 mg/lb BW PO sid daily for heartworm prevention (Kinsell, 1986)
     25-50 mg/lb BW PO once, repeat in 10-20 days for ascarids (Kinsell, 1986)

N   50 mg/kg sid × 10 days in orange juice (Eberhard, 1982)

Diiodohydroxyquin

N   20 mg/kg BW PO bid for three weeks (Russell et al, 1981)
     30 mg/kg BW PO for 10 days (Cummins et al, 1973)
     630 mg/chimpanzee PO tid for 3 weeks (Van Riper et al, 1966)
     650 mg daily per animal PO for 10-20 days (Ialeggio, 1989)

Dimetridazole (no longer available)

H   1 g/L drinking water for 2 weeks (La Regina et al, 1980)

M   1 g/L drinking water for 2 weeks (Frost, 1977)
     10 mg/ml drinking water for 5 days (Roach et al, 1988)

Dithiazanine iodide

M   0.1 mg/g food for 7 days (Williams, 1976)

N   10-20 mg/kg BW PO sid for 3-10 days (Russell et al, 1981)
     100 mg/12-20 lb BW bid for 2 weeks (maple syrup acts as vehicle) (Van Riper et al, 1966)

Re 20 mg/kg BW PO sid for 10 days (Frye, 1981)

Emetine hydrochloride

Re 0.5 mg/kg BW/day IM, SC sid, bid for 10 days (Frye, 1981)

Fenbendazole

Am 10 mg/kg BW PO (Cooper, 1985)

Bi 20-50 mg/kg BW PO once each week for 2 weeks for ascarids (Nemetz, 1990)

20-50 mg/kg BW PO sid for 5 days for capillaria (Not always effective) (Nemetz, 1990)

Note: Do not use while bird is nesting

Bo 7.5 mg/kg BW PO (Schultz, 1989)

C 33 mg/kg BW PO sid for 5-7 days (Kinsell, 1986)

D 50 mg/kg BW PO sid for 3 days (Kinsell, 1986)

Go 5 mg/kg BW PO (Schultz, 1989)

M 100 ppm in the food for 14 days (Reiss et al, 1987)

20 mg/kg BW PO for 5 days (McKellar, 1989)

N *Lemur, Varecia:* 50 mg/kg BW PO sid for 3 days (Feeser and White, 1992)

R 8-12 mg/kg BW/day in feed daily (150 ppm) on alternating weeks (Coghlan et al, 1993)

20 mg/kg BW PO for 5 days (McKellar, 1989)

Rb 50 ppm in the food for 5 days (Duwel and Brech, 1981)

20 mg/kg BW PO for 5 days (McKellar, 1989)

Rc 50 mg/kg BW PO sid for 3 days (Evans and Evans, 1986)

Re Tortoises: 50-100 mg/kg BW PO once; repeat in 2 weeks (Page and Mautino, 1990)

Sh 5 mg/kg BW PO (Schultz, 1989)

Sw 5 mg/kg BW PO (Schultz, 1989)

Furadantin—*See* nitrofurantoin

Iodoquinol—*See* diiodohydroxyquin

Ipronidazole (no longer available)

Bi 500 mg (0.25 tsp)/gal water for 7 days. Drug of choice for proto-zoan disease in psittacines (Nemetz, 1990)

Ivermectin

Am *Rana pipiens:* 2 mg/kg BW SC (Letcher and Glade, 1992)

Bi 0.2 mg/kg BW PO, IM, or percutaneously over right jugular vein.

Note: Add 0.1 ml 1% ivermectin to 9.9 ml sterile water. Resulting solution is 0.1 mg/ml. To dose a 50-g bird use 10 μg (0.1 ml) of dilution (Schultz, 1989; Nemetz, 1990)

Bo 0.2 mg/kg BW SC (Schultz, 1989)
F 1 mg/kg BW SC total dose (Egerton et al, 1980)
Gp 500 μg/kg BW SC (McKellar et al, 1992)
M 2 mg/kg BW given by gavage, repeat in 10 days
    1 part 1% ivermectin with 10 parts tap water. Mist 1-2 mls over entire cage (Le Blanc et al, 1993)
N 200 μg/kg BW IM, repeat in 10 days (Battles et al, 1988)
    200 μg/kg BW SC (Ialeggio, 1989)
    200 μg/kg BW PO (Feeser and White, 1992)
R 200 μg/kg BW sid for 5 days by gastric intubation (Battles et al, 1987)
    200 μg/kg BW SC once (Findon and Miller, 1987)
    3 mg/kg BW PO once (Summa er al, 1992)
    2 mg/kg BW PO for 3 treatments at 7-9 day intervals (Huerkamp, 1993)
Rb 400 μg/kg BW SC (McKellar et al, 1992)
Sw 0.3 mg/kg BW SC (Schultz, 1989)

Levamisole

Am 10 mg/kg BW IM (Cooper, 1985)
Bi 10-20 mg/kg BW IM, repeat in 2 weeks; emesis common, may be toxic (Nemetz, 1990)
    10 ml of 13.65%/gal water as only source for 1-3 days; repeat in 10 days (Nemetz, 1990)
    4-8 mg/kg BW IM once; repeat in 10-14 days (Harrison and Harrison, 1986)
Bo 8 mg/kg BW SC, PO (Schultz, 1989)
N 7.5 mg/kg BW SC, repeat in 2 weeks (Welshman, 1985)
Rc 4-10 mg/kg BW PO (Evans and Evans, 1986)
Re 5 mg/kg BW intracoelomic once, may be repeated in 2-3 weeks (Frye, 1981)
Sh 3 mg/kg BW SC, PO (Schultz, 1989)
Sw 8 mg/kg BW SC, PO (Schultz, 1989)

Lime sulfur

Gp 1:40 sponged over body weekly for 6 weeks (Russell et al, 1981)

Lindane

Gp 1% used as a dip (Zajac et al, 1980)
M 0.25% dust (Hawk, 1991)
R 0.25% dust (Hawk, 1991)

Malathion

Gp 0.5% used as a dip (Russell et al, 1981)
M 5 ml of 1% suspension in bedding (Russell et al, 1981)
R 5 ml of 1% suspension in bedding (Russell et al, 1981)
Rb 0.5% sponged twice weekly (Russell et al, 1981)

Mebendazole

Bi 40-60 mg/kg PO once (Nemetz, 1990)
    25 mg/kg BW bid for 5 days (Harrison and Harrison, 1986)
D 10 mg active ingredient/lb BW PO sid sprinkled on food for 5 days,
    may repeat in 3 weeks (Kinsell, 1986)
G 2.2 mg/ml tap water/animal sid for 5 days, by gavage (Smith and
    Snider, 1988)
M 40 mg/kg BW as a drench, repeat in 7 days (Russell et al, 1981)
N 3-5 mg/kg BW PO (Russell et al, 1981)
    15 mg/kg BW PO for 3 days (Wolff, 1990)
    22 mg/kg BW PO sid for 3 days, repeat in 2 weeks.
R 10 mg/kg BW PO for 5 days (McKellar, 1989)
Rb 10 mg/kg BW PO for 5 days (McKellar, 1989)
Rc 25-40 mg/kg BW PO sid for 3-5 days (Evans and Evans, 1986)

Metyridine

R 125 mg/kg BW SC once (Weisbroth and Scher, 1971)
    125 mg/kg BW IP once (Weisbroth and Scher, 1971)
    200 mg/kg BW IP once (Peardon et al, 1966)

Metronidazole

Bi Lovebirds: 10 mg/kg BW IM sid for 3 days (Nemetz, 1990)
    Cockatiels: 35-50 mg/kg BW IM sid for 5 days; repeat in 2-4 weeks
    (Nemetz, 1990)
D 60 mg/kg BW PO sid for 5 days (Kinsell, 1986)
F 35 mg/kg BW PO sid for 5 days (Bell, 1994)
Gp 20 mg/kg BW PO, SC sid (Richardson, 1992)
M 2.5 mg/ml drinking water for 5 days (Roach et al, 1988)

N   35-50 mg/kg/day BW PO bid for 10 days (Holmes, 1984)
Re 125-275 mg/kg BW PO once, may be repeated at 7-10 day intervals
        for 1-2 more treatments (Frye, 1981)
        Tortoises: 250 mg/kg BW PO once, repeat in 2 weeks (Page and
        Mautino, 1990)

Niclosamide

Bi 220 mg/kg BW PO once; repeat in 10-14 days (Harrison and
        Harrison, 1986)
        Finches—500 mg/kg BW PO once a week for 4 weeks (Harrison
        and Harrison, 1986)
G   1 mg/10 g BW PO (Burke, 1979)
H   500 mg in 150 g food (Burke, 1979)
        10 mg/100 g BW PO as a drench, repeat in 2 weeks (Russell et al,
        1981)
M   100 mg/kg BW once PO (Harkness and Wagner, 1983)
        500 mg/150 g ground feed for 1 week (Williams, 1976)
N   30 mg/kg BW PO, repeat in 2-3 weeks (Russell et al, 1976)
        140 mg/kg BW PO (Williams, 1976)
R   100 mg/kg BW once PO (Harkness and Wagner, 1983)
        10 mg/100 g BW as a drench, repeat in 2 weeks (Russell et al, 1981)
        1 mg/g feed for two weeks seperated by 1 week (Russell et al, 1981)
Rb 150 mg/kg BW PO (Williams, 1976)
Re 150 mg/kg BW PO, not more often than once each month (Frye,
        1981)

Nitrofurantoin

R   0.2% in feed for 6-8 weeks (Russell et al, 1981)

Paromomycin

N   50 mg/kg BW PO in 3 divided doses sid for 10 days (Williams,
        1976)

Phenothiazine

Rb 1 g/50 g molasses treated feed (Merck Veterinary Manual, 1979)

Piperazine (adipate and citrate)

Bi 250-500 mg/kg BW PO once, repeat in 2 weeks (Nemetz, 1990)

Bo 110 mg/kg BW PO (Schultz, 1989)

C 0.86 g/lb BW PO, repeat in 10-21 days (Kinsell, 1986)

D 0.86 g/lb BW PO, repeat in 10-21 days (Kinsell, 1986)

G 20-60 mg/100 g BW PO (Russell et al, 1981)

    3-5 mg/ml drinking water for 7 days, off 7 days, repeat for 7 days (Russell et al, 1981)

Go 110 mg/kg BW PO (Schultz, 1989)

Gp Piperazine adipate—4-7 mg/ml in drinking water (Williams, 1976)

H 3-5 mg/ml drinking water for 7 days, off 7 days, repeat for 7 days (Russell et al, 1981)

    Piperazine citrate—10 mg/ml drinking water for 7 days, off 5 days, repeat for 7 days (Unay and Davis, 1980)

    Piperazine citrate—2 ml of 10 mg/ml given once by gavage (Unay and Davis, 1980)

M 500 mg/100 ml drinking water for 14 days (Reiss et al, 1987)

    Piperazine adipate—4-7 mg/ml drinking water for 3-10 days (Williams, 1976)

    Piperazine citrate—200 mg/kg BW daily in drinking water for 7 consecutive days, off 7 days, then repeat for another 7 consecutive days (Hoag, 1961)

N 65 mg/kg BW PO sid for 10 days (Russell et al, 1981)

    100 mg/kg BW PO (Ialeggio, 1989)

R 200 mg/100 ml drinking water (Rossof, 1974)

    Piperazine adipate—250 mg/50-60 g BW in drinking water for three days (Habermann and Williams, 1957)

    Piperazine adipate—50 mg/ml in drinking water for 3 days (Hawk, 1991)

    Piperazine citrate—4 g/L drinking water for 7 days, off 7 days, repeat for 7 days (Hawk, 1991)

Rb Piperazine adipate—0.5 mg/kg BW PO for 2 days (Brooks, 1979)

    Piperazine citrate—100 mg/ml drinking water for 1 day (USDA, 1976)

    Piperazine powder—200 mg/kg BW PO (Harkness and Wagner, 1983)

Rc 75-150 mg/kg PO (Evans and Evans, 1986)

Re Piperazine citrate—40-60 mg/kg BW PO, not more often than once every 2 weeks (Frye, 1981)

Sh 110 mg/kg BW PO (Schultz, 1989)

Sw 110 mg/kg BW PO (Schultz, 1989)

Praziquantel
Bi 6 mg/kg BW PO once; toxic to finches (Nemetz, 1990)
     9-16 mg/kg BW IM once; toxic to finches (Nemetz, 1990)
M 5 mg/kg BW sc or 10 mg/kg BW PO (McKellar, 1989)
N 0.1 ml/kg BW IM (Droncit injectable) (Welshman, 1985)
     40 mg/kg BW PO, IM once (Wolff, 1990)
R 5 mg/kg BW sc or 10 mg/kg BW PO (McKellar, 1989)
Rb 5 mg/kg BW sc or 10 mg/kg BW PO (McKellar, 1989)
Rc 5-10 mg/kg BW IM, PO (Evans and Evans, 1986)
     10-15 mg/kg BW SC, may be given up to 100 mg/kg BW for some
        trematodes (Evans and Evans, 1986)

Pyrantel pamoate
Bi 4.5 mg/kg BW PO sid, repeat in 2 weeks (Nemetz, 1990)
D 1 ml/5-20 lb BW PO (Kinsell, 1986)
N *Lemur:* 6 mg/kg BW PO (Feeser and White, 1992)
Rc 10-20 mg/kg BW PO (Evans and Evans, 1986)

Pyrethrin
Rb 0.5% applied as a dust (Russell, 1981)

Pyrvinium pamoate
H 0.8 mg/L drinking water for 30 days (Frost, 1977)
M 0.8 mg/L drinking water for 28 days (Russell et al, 1981)
N 5 mg/kg BW PO every 6 months (more often if needed) (Cummins
       et al, 1973)
R 0.003% in drinking water for 30 days (Blair and Thompson, 1969)
     0.012% in food for 30 days (Blair and Thompson, 1969)

Quinacrine hydrochloride
Bi 5-10 mg/kg BW PO sid for 7 days (Harrison and Harrison, 1986)
N 10 mg/kg BW PO tid every 10 days (Russell et al, 1981)
R 75 mg/kg BW PO total dose (Balazs et al, 1962)

Ronnel
Gp 45 ml of 33 ⅓% suspension in 250 ml propylene glycol

N   55 mg/kg BW PO every other day × 4 treatments, then once weekly for 3 months; a total of 16 treatments (Finegold et al, 1968)

Rotenone

Bi   Apply cream once each week for 4 weeks (Nemetz, 1990)

Note: Ivermectin is the drug of choice.

N   One part rotenone in 3 parts mineral oil applied topically once a week for two weeks (Bowman and Griffith, 1987)
Rb   Mix with mineral oil and apply in ear for 3 days off and on for 3 weeks (Russell, 1981)

Tetrachlorethylene

Re   0.2 ml/kg BW PO, not more often than once each month (Frye, 1981)

Thiabendazole

Bi   250-500 mg/kg BW PO once, repeat in 2 weeks (Nemetz, 1990)
Bo   66 mg/kg BW PO, 110 mg/kg BW PO for severe parasitism and *Cooperia* (Schultz, 1989)
M   100-200 mg/kg BW PO (Harkness and Wagner, 1983)
N   50-100 mg/kg BW PO, repeat in 2 weeks (Van Riper et al, 1966)
        100 mg/kg BW PO, repeat in 2 weeks, then once every 6 months (Cummins et al, 1973; Ialeggio, 1989)
        100 mg/kg BW PO sid for 3 days (Welshman, 1985)
R   200 mg/kg BW PO for 5 days (Rossof, 1974)
        0.1% in the feed (Harkness and Wagner, 1983)
Rb   25 mg/kg BW PO (Williams, 1976)
        100 mg/kg BW PO for 5 days (McKellar, 1989)
Re   50 mg/kg BW PO as a drench, use as often as necessary (Frye, 1981)
Sw   75 mg/kg BW PO (Schultz, 1989)

Thiabendazole and piperazine hydrate

H   0.1% thiabendazole in the diet for 6 weeks, and 0.6% piperazine in the drinking water starting two weeks before the thiabendazole (Taylor, 1992)

Tinidazole

M   2.5 mg/ml drinking water for 5 days (Roach et al, 1988)

Trichlorfon

M   1.75 g/L drinking water with 1 g sugar, for 14 days, assuming a
         mouse consumes 2.2-3.2 ml water daily (Simmons et al, 1965)
         175 mg/100 ml drinking water for 14 days (Reiss et al, 1987)

Vapona pest strip (DDVP). *See also* Dichlorvos, 48-49

M   Place a 1 × 1 inch strip on each cage (for 24 hours) on cage chang-
         ing day for four changings (our interpretation of French, 1987,
         Eds.)
Re   1 strip/1000 cu. ft. room space, use continuously (Frye, 1981)

MISCELLANEOUS DRUGS

Acetylcysteine

M   653 mg/kg PO IP (Borchard et al, 1990)
      1200 mg/kg BW PO (Borchard et al, 1990)
R   400 mg/kg BW IP (Borchard et al, 1990)

Allopurinol

Bi 10 mg/oz drinking water (Nemetz, 1990)
      30 mg/kg BW PO (Nemetz, 1990)
D   10 mg/kg BW PO q8h, then reduce to 10 mg/kg BW PO sid
      (Kinsell, 1986)

Alloxan

C   1 ml of a 10% solution in citrate-phosphate buffer (pH 3.5-4.0)
      given IA at a rate of 0.5 ml/min (Reiser et al,1987)
      750 mg/kg BW PO (Borchard et al, 1990)
M 75 mg/kg BW IV (Borchard et al, 1990)
R   40 mg/kg BW IV (Borchard et al, 1990)
      200 mg/kg BW IP, SC (Borchard et al, 1990)

Aminophylline

Bi 3.75 mg/macaw BID (Nemetz, 1990)
C   10 mg/kg BW IM, IV q18-12h: for IV use, dilute in 10-20 ml
      normal saline or 5% dextrose in water and inject slowly (Kinsell,
      1986)

D   10 mg/kg BW IM, IV q18-12h: for IV use, dilute in 10-20 ml normal saline or 5% dextrose in water and inject slowly (Kinsell, 1986)

N   25-100 mg/animal PO bid (Johnson et al, 1981)
Lemur: 10 mg/kg BW IV (Feeser and White, 1992)

Re   2-4 mg/kg BW IM as needed (Frye, 1981)

Amitriptyline

C   5-10 mg total dose PO (Borchard et al, 1990)
D   1-2 mg/kg BW PO (Borchard et al, 1990)
M   1 mg/kg BW IP, PO (Borchard et al, 1990)
R   20 mg/kg BW IP (Borchard et al, 1990)
10 mg/kg BW SC (Borchard et al, 1990)
30 mg/kg BW PO (Borchard et al, 1990)

Amphetamine

M   5 mg/kg BW IP (Taber and Irwin, 1969)

Atropine

Bi   0.04-0.01 mg/kg BW IM, SC (Harrison and Harrison, 1986)
0.1-0.2 mg/kg BW IM, SC for organophosphate overdose (Harrison and Harrison, 1986)

Bo   0.6-0.12 mg/kg BW IV (Schultz, 1989)
0.5-1.0 mg/kg BW IV, may repeat in 1-2 hours; for organophosphate poisoning (Schultz, 1989)

C   0.05 mg/kg BW IM, IV, SC q6h (Kinsell, 1986)
Ch   0.15 mg/kg BW SC, IM, IV (Rossoff, 1974)
D   0.05 mg/kg BW IM, IV, SC q6h (Kinsell, 1986)
F   0.05 mg/kg BW IM, SC (Andrews and Illman, 1987)
G   0.02-0.05 mg/kg BW SC, IM, IV (CCAC, 1984)
Go   0.04-0.80 mg/kg BW IM (Swindle and Adams, 1988)
0.13 mg/kg BW IV (Swindle and Adams, 1988)
Gp   0.02-0.05 mg/kg SC, IM, IV (CCAC, 1984)
H   0.02-0.05 mg/kg BW SC, IM, IV (CCAC, 1984)
M   0.05 mg/kg BW IM, SC, IV (Green, 1982)
0.02-0.05 mg/kg BW SC, IM, IV (CCAC, 1984)
N   0.10 mg/kg BW SC (Domino et al, 1969)
0.05 mg/kg BW SC, IM, IV (CCAC, 1984)
R   0.04 mg/kg BW IM (Weisbroth and Fudens, 1972)
0.02-0.05 mg/kg BW SC, IM, IV (CCAC, 1984)

Rb 0.20 mg/kg BW IM, IV, SC (Green, 1982)

10 mg/kg BW SC every 20 min for organophosphate overdose (Harkness and Wagner, 1983)

1-3 mg/kg BW IM, SC 30 min before surgery (Green, 1982)

Re 0.04 mg/kg BW IM, IV, SC, PO as needed (Frye, 1981)

Sh 0.04-0.80 mg/kg BW IM (Swindle and Adams, 1988)

0.13 mg/kg BW IV (Swindle and Adams, 1988)

Sw 0.05-0.5 mg/kg BW SC (Swindle and Adams, 1988)

0.044-0.4 mg/kg BW IM (Swindle and Adams, 1988)

Betamethasone

Gp 0.1-0.2 ml IM, SC (Richarson, 1992)

Bretylium

C 15 mg/kg BW IV (Borchard et al, 1990)

D 5 mg/kg BW IV (Borchard et al, 1990)

M 12.5 mg/kg BW IV (Borchard et al, 1990)

N 200 mg/kg BW PO (Borchard et al, 1990)

R 5 mg/kg BW IV (Borchard et al, 1990)

400 mg/kg BW PO (Borchard et al, 1990)

Rb 10 mg/kg BW IV (Borchard et al, 1990)

Sw 5 mg/kg BW IV (Schumann et al, 1993)

Bromhexine

Bi 0.15 mg/100 g BW IM bid, sid (Harrison and Harrison, 1986)

Calcium borogluconate

Re 10 ml/kg BW of 1% solution IM, SC (Bennett, 1989)

Calcium EDTA

Bi 35 mg/kg BW IM bid, tid for 5-7 days, then switch to oral form (Nemetz, 1990)

Bo 110 mg/kg BW IP, IM in 1-2% solution in 5% glucose. Skip 2 days and repeat for 2 days for up to 10-14 days (Schultz, 1989)

Calcium gluconate—*Also see* Calphosan

Bi 50-100 mg/kg BW IM, IV [slow] (Nemetz, 1990)

Calphosan (calcium gluconate/calcium lactate)

Bi   0.5-1 ml/kg BW IM once, can repeat weekly (Harrison and Harrison, 1986)

Chloroquine phosphate

N   Rhesus monkey: 150 mg/adult PO day 1 and 3 (Schofield et al, 1985)

Chlorpheniramine

Gp   5 mg/kg BW SC (Borchard et al, 1990)
M   1 mg/kg BW IP (Borchard et al, 1990)
N   0.5 mg/kg BW/day PO in divided doses (Johnson et al, 1981)

Chlorpromazine

C   1-2 mg/kg BW IV, IM q12h (Kinsell, 1986)
D   1.1-6.6 mg/kg BW IM q6-24h (Kinsell, 1986)
   0.55-4.4 mg/kg BW IV q6-12h (Kinsell, 1986)
G   0.5 mg/kg BW IM (CCAC, 1984)
Go   2.2 mg/kg BW PO (Swindle and Adams, 1988)
   1.0-4.4 mg/kg BW IM (Swindle and Adams, 1988)
   0.22-1.10 mg/kg BW IV (Swindle and Adams, 1988)
Gp   0.5 mg/kg BW IM (CCAC, 1984)
H   0.5 mg/kg BW IM (Melby and Altman, 1976)
M   3-5 mg/kg BW IV or 3-35 mg/kg BW IM (Harkness and Wagner, 1983)
N   1-3 mg/kg BW IM (Melby and Altman, 1976)
   2-5 mg/kg BW PO (CCAC, 1984)
R   3-5 mg/kg BW IV or 3-35 mg/kg BW IM (Harkness and Wagner, 1983)
Sh   2.2 mg/kg BW PO (Swindle and Adams, 1988)
   1-4.4 mg/kg BW IM (Swindle and Adams, 1988)
   0.22-1.10 mg/kg BW IV (Swindle and Adams, 1988)
Sw   0.5-4.0 mg/kg BW IM (Swindle and Adams, 1988)
   0.55-3.3 mg/kg BW IV (Swindle and Adams, 1988)

Cholestyramine (for reversal of antibiotic-induced enterocolitis)

Rb   Cholestyramine (2 g active ingredient which is equivalent to 4 g of of Questran™) in 20 ml drinking water for 21 days Lipman et al, 1989)

Cortisone

R   0.25-1.25 mg/day SC, IM, PO (Rossoff, 1974)

Dexamethasone

Bo 5-20 mg IV, IM, PO (Schultz, 1989)
C   0.125-0.5 mg sid or divided doses IV, IM, PO (Kinsell, 1986)
D   0.25-1.25 mg sid or divided bid PO (Kinsell, 1986)
      0.25-1.0 mg sid IM, IV (Kinsell, 1986)
Gp 0.1 ml SC (Richardson, 1992)
N   0.25-1.0 mg/kg BW PO, IM total dose (Melby and Altman, 1976)
Re 0.625-0.125 mg/kg BW IV, IM as needed (Frye, 1981)

Dexamethasone sodium phosphate

Bi 2-8 mg/kg BW IM, IV for shock, endotoxemia (Nemetz, 1990)
Bo 1-2 mg/kg BW slow IV (Schultz, 1989)
C   1-5 mg/kg BW slow IV (Schultz, 1989)
D   1-5 mg/kg BW slow IV (Schultz, 1989)
Sh 1-2 mg/kg BW slow IV (Schultz, 1989)

Diethylstilbestrol

Bi 0.03-0.1 ml of 0.25 mg/ml stock per 30 g BW IM (Harrison and Harrison, 1986)
      1 drop of 0.25 mg/ml stock per 30 ml drinking water (Harrison and Harrison, 1986)
C   0.05-0.1 mg/day PO (Kinsell, 1986)
D   0.1-1 mg/day PO (Kinsell, 1986)

Dimethyl sulfoxide

Bi 0.1 ml/100 g BW topical or nebulization (Nemetz, 1990)
D   Apply topically. Do not exceed 20 ml per day for 14 days (Kinsell, 1986)

Diphenhydramine

C   4 mg/kg BW PO q8h (Kinsell, 1986)
      0.5 mg/lb BW IV (considered a high dose by Kinsell, 1986)
D   4 mg/kg BW PO q8h (Kinsell, 1986)
      0.5 mg/lb BW IV (considered a high dose by Kinsell, 1986)

Gp 5 mg/kg BW SC (Melby and Altman, 1976)
    12.5 mg/kg BW IP (Borchard et al, 1990)
M 50 mg/kg BW IP (Borchard et al, 1990)
N *Lemur:* 5 mg/kg BW IM (Feeser and White, 1992)
R 10 mg/kg BW SC (Borchard et al, 1990)

Diphenoxylate and atropine sulfate

N 1 ml/animal PO tid (Holmes, 1984)

Docusate sodium

Bi 10 mg/oz drinking water (Nemetz, 1990)

Doxapram

Bi 5-10 mg/kg BW IV, IM once (Harrison and Harrison, 1986)
C 5-10 mg/kg BW IV, may repeat in 15-20 min (Kinsell, 1986)
D 5-10 mg/kg BW IV, may repeat in 15-20 min (Kinsell, 1986)
F 1-2 mg/kg BW IV (Flecknell, 1987)
G 5-10 mg/kg BW IV (Flecknell, 1987)
Go 2-10 mg/kg BW IV (Swindle and Adams, 1988)
Gp 5 mg/kg BW IV (Flecknell, 1987)
    10-15 mg/kg BW IM, SC (Richardson, 1992)
H 5-10 mg/kg BW IV (Flecknell, 1987)
M 5-10 mg/kg BW IV (Flecknell, 1987)
N 2 mg/kg BW IV (Flecknell, 1987)
R 5-10 mg/kg BW IV (Flecknell, 1987)
Rb 2-5 mg/kg BW IV (Flecknell, 1987)
Sh 2-10 mg/kg BW IV (Swindle and Adams, 1988)
Sw 2-10 mg/kg BW IV (Swindle and Adams, 1988)

Enalapril

D 0.5 mg/kg BW PO sid (Package insert)

Furosemide

Bi 0.05 mg/300 g BW IM bid (Harrison and Harrison, 1986)
C 2 mg/kg BW IV q12h to a maximum total dose of 5 mg (Kinsell, 1986)
    2-4 mg/kg PO q8-12h (Kinsell, 1986)

D 2 mg/kg BW IV q12h to a maximum total dose of 40 mg (Kinsell, 1986)

2-4 mg/kg PO q8-12h (Kinsell, 1986)

N 2 mg/kg BW PO (Johnson et al, 1981)

Re 5 mg/kg BW IM, IV sid or bid (Frye, 1981)

Gallamine

Am 6 mg/kg BW in ventral lymph sac (Lumb and Jones, 1984)

M 1.2 mg/kg BW IV (Lumb and Jones, 1984)

R 0.01 mg/kg BW IV (Borchard et al, 1990)

Rb 0.2-0.3 mg/kg BW IV (Lumb and Jones, 1984)

Glycopyrrolate

C 5 µg/lb or 0.25 ml/10 lb BW IM (Package insert)

N 13-17 µg/kg IM (Sanders et al, 1991)

Heparin

C 1 mg/kg BW IV (Kinsell, 1986)

D 1 mg/kg BW IV (Kinsell, 1986)

Gp 5 mg/kg BW IV (Melby and Altman, 1976)

M 10 mg/kg BW IV (Melby and Altman, 1976)

N 2 mg/kg BW IV (Melby and Altman, 1976)

R 10 mg/kg BW IV (Borchard et al, 1990)

Rb 5 mg/kg BW IV (Melby and Altman, 1976)

Indapamide

R 3 mg/kg BW IP (Delbarre and Delbarre, 1988)

Insulin

N Start NPH at 0.25-0.5 units/kg BW/day SC (Schultz, 1989)

Iodine (Lugol's)

Bi 2 ml/30 ml water stock. Dose at 1 drop in each 250 ml water given daily for goiter (Harrison and Harrison, 1986)

Iron dextran

Bi   10 mg/kg BW IM, repeat weekly (Harrison and Harrison, 1986)

Kaolin

Gp   0.2 ml given 3-4 times daily (Kaopectate V) (Richardson, 1992)

Kaolin and pectin

N   0.5-1 ml/kg BW PO q2-6h (Johnson et al, 1981)

Levallorphan

Any species: give 1 mg Levallorphan (up to a maximum of 0.5 mg/kg BW) for every 50 mg of morphine that was given (Green, 1982)

Levonorgestrel

N   1 mg/kg BW PO q24h (Mann et al, 1986)

Levothyroxine

Bi   0.1 mg/30-120 ml water (Nemetz, 1990)

Loperamide

Rb   0.1 mg/kg BW PO tid for 3 days, then sid for 2 days (Banerjee et al, 1987)

Medroxyprogesterone acetate

Bi   30 mg/kg BW SC every 6 weeks to 3 months (Nemetz, 1990)

Note: Check for lipoma development.

Re   20 mg/kg BW IM (Bennett, 1989)

Meprobamate

Gp   100 mg/kg BW IM (Melby and Altman, 1976)
H   100 mg/kg BW IM (Melby and Altman, 1976)
M   100 mg/kg BW IM (Melby and Altman, 1976)
N   100-400 mg/kg BW PO (Melby and Altman, 1976)

R   150 mg/kg BW IM (Melby and Altman, 1976)
Rb 50-150 mg/kg BW IM (Melby and Altman, 1976)

Methylprednisone

C   1 mg/kg BW IM per week (Kinsell, 1986)
D   20 mg or less intrasynovially (Kinsell, 1986)
        1 mg/kg BW IM per week (Kinsell, 1986)
Gp 2 mg/kg BW IM every 30 days (Bauck, 1989)

Metocurine

Am 0.94 mg/kg BW in ventral lymph sac (Lumb and Jones, 1984)
M   0.08-0.1 mg/kg BW IV (Lumb and Jones, 1984)
R   0.009 mg/kg BW IV (Lumb and Jones, 1984)
Rb 0.01-0.015 mg/kg BW IV (Lumb and Jones, 1984)

Mineral oil

Bi 1-3 drops/ 30 g BW PO once (Harrison and Harrison, 1986)
        5 ml/kg BW PO once (Harrison and Harrison, 1986)
C   2-6 ml PO (Kinsell, 1986)
D   5-30 ml PO (Kinsell, 1986)

Nalorphine

Note: Any species: give 1 mg Nalorphine (up to a maximum of 2 mg/kg BW) for every 10 mg of morphine that was given. (Green, 1982)

C   1 mg/kg BW IM, IV, SC. No more than 5 mg per dose (Kinsell, 1986)
D   5 mg/kg BW IM, IV, SC. No more than 5 mg per dose (Kinsell, 1986)
M   2 mg/kg BW IV (Harkness and Wagner, 1983)
R   2 mg/kg BW IV (Harkness and Wagner, 1983)
Rb 2 mg/kg BW IV (Harkness and Wagner, 1983)

Naloxone

D   Dose to effect, usually 0.2-0.4 mg total dose IM, SC, IV (Kinsell, 1986)
G   0.01-0.1 mg/kg BW IP, IV (Flecknell, 1987)
Gp 0.01-0.1 mg/kg BW IP, IV (Flecknell, 1987)

H   0.01-0.1 mg/kg BW IP, IV (Flecknell, 1987)
M   0.01-0.1 mg/kg BW IP, IV (Flecknell, 1987)
N   0.01-0.05 mg/kg BW IM, IV (Flecknell, 1987)
        2-3 ml SC, IM, IV (Rosenberg, 1991)
R   0.01-0.1 mg/kg BW IP, IV (Flecknell, 1987)
Rb 0.01-0.1 mg/kg BW IM, IV (Flecknell, 1987)

Oxytocin

Bi 0.2-2 units IM (Nemetz, 1990)

Note: Always give parenteral calcium and vitamin A at least 10 min before oxytocin.

Bo 75-100 units IM, IV (Schultz, 1989)
C   5-10 units IM, IV, SC (Kinsell, 1986)
D   5-30 units IM, IV, SC (Kinsell, 1986)
Gp 1-2 units IM (Richardson, 1992)
N   5-20 units IM, IV total dose (Melby and Altman, 1976)
R   1 unit SC, IM total dose (Rossoff, 1974)
Rb 1-2 units IM, SC total dose (Melby and Altman, 1976)
Re 1-10 units/kg BW IM (Bennett, 1989)
Sh 30-50 units IM, IV, SC (Kinsell, 1986)
Sw 30-50 units IM, IV, SC (Kinsell, 1986)

Pancuronium

C   0.1 mg/kg BW IV (Borchard et al, 1990)
D   0.1 mg/kg BW IV (Borchard et al, 1990)
M   0.03 mg/kg BW IV (Lumb and Jones, 1984)
Rb 0.008 mg/kg BW IV (Lumb and Jones, 1984)

Prednisolone

C   For prolonged use, 2-4 mg/kg BW PO qod (Kinsell, 1986)
        For immune suppression, 3 mg/kg BW IM, PO q12h (Kinsell, 1986)
        For allergy, 1 mg/kg BW IM, PO q12h (Kinsell, 1986)
D   For prolonged use, 0.5-2 mg/kg BW PO qod (Kinsell, 1986)
        For immune suppression, 2 mg/kg BW IM, PO q12h (Kinsell, 1986)
        For allergy, 0.5 mg/kg BW IM, PO q12h (Kinsell, 1986)

Prednisolone sodium succinate

Bi 10-20 mg/kg BW IV, IM every 15 min to effect (Harrison and Harrison, 1986)

D 5.5-11 mg/kg BW IV, then repeat at 1, 3, 6, or 10 h prn (Kinsell, 1986)

N 1-15 mg/kg BW PO total dose (Melby and Altman, 1976)
1-5 mg/kg BW/day PO (Rosenberg et al, 1987)
10 mg/kg BW IV (Feeser and White, 1992)
Lemur: 10 mg/kg BW IV (Feeser and White, 1992)

Re 5-10 mg/kg BW IM, IV as needed (Frye, 1981)

Prednisone

N 0.5-1 mg/kg BW PO bid for 3-5 days, then sid for 3-5 days, then q48h for 10 days, then one-half dose q48h (Isaza et al, 1992)

Scopolamine

N 0.01 mg/kg BW SC (Domino et al, 1969)

Stanozolol—*See* Winstrol-V

Streptozotocin

M 200 mg/kg BW IV once (Fromtling et al, 1985)

N 45-55 mg/kg BW IV once (Takimoto et al, 1988)

R 55 mg/kg BW IV (Borchard et al, 1990)
60 mg/kg BW IP (Borchard et al, 1990)
22 mg/kg BW IM (Borchard et al, 1990)
50 mg/kg BW IP (Alder et al, 1992)

Succinylcholine

Am 2.5 mg/kg BW in ventral lymph sac (Lumb and Jones,1984)

C 0.06 mg/kg BW via continuous IV infusion (Kinsell, 1986)

D 0.07 mg/kg BW via continuous IV infusion (Kinsell, 1986)

M 0.05-0.1 mg/kg BW IV (Lumb and Jones, 1984)

N 2 mg/kg BW IV (USAF, 1976)

Rb 0.5 mg/kg BW IV (Green, 1982)

Re Chelonians: 0.25-1.5 mg/kg BW IM (Page, 1993)

Sh 0.02 mg/kg BW via continuous IV infusion (Kinsell, 1986)
Sw 0.12-0.18 mg/kg BW via continuous IV infusion (PUSVM,1986)

Testosterone

Bi Canary—Stock: 100 mg/oz water. Dose: use 5 drops/oz drinking water for 1-2 months [to finish molt or to regain singing] (Nemetz, 1990)
8.5 mg/kg BW IM once, then weekly as needed (Nemetz, 1990)

Tolazoline

Bo 0.2 mg/kg BW IV (Schultz, 1989)
0.5 mg/kg BW SC (Schultz, 1989)
Go 2-5 mg/kg BW IV slowly over 1 minute (NCSU, 1987)
Sh 2-5 mg/kg BW IV slowly over 1 minute (NCSU, 1987)

Tripelennamine

Gp 5 mg/kg BW PO, IM (Melby and Altman, 1976)

Tubocurarine

Am 1.4-7.5 mg/kg BW in ventral lymph sac (Lumb and Jones,1984)
M 0.06-0.09 mg/kg BW IV (Lumb and Jones, 1984)
N 0.09 mg/kg BW IV (USAF, 1976)
R 0.04-0.06 mg/kg BW IV (Lumb and Jones, 1984)
Rb 0.09-0.15 mg/kg BW IV (Lumb and Jones, 1984)

Vitamin A

Bi 100,000 IU/kg BW IM two times the first week, then once weekly (Nemetz, 1990)

Note: If using Injacom Plus® (contains B-complex), do not exceed 3 mg thiamine/100 g bird.

Re 50,000 IU every 2 weeks IM (Snipes, 1984)
Tortoises: 11,000 IU/kg BW IM once (Page and Mautino,1990)

Vitamin B complex

Bi 10-30 mg/kg IM bid to once each week [dose on thiamine content; do not exceed 3 mg thiamine/100 g bird] (Nemetz, 1990)

C 1-2 ml IM, IV, 1-2 times per week prn (Kinsell, 1986)

D 1-2 ml Im, IV, 1-2 times per week prn (Kinsell, 1986)

Vitamin C

Bi 20-40 mg/kg IM sid to once each week (Harrison and Harrison, 1986)

C 100 mg/day PO (Kinsell, 1986)
25-75 mg IM, IV, SC (Kinsell, 1986)
100 mg PO q8h as urinary acidifier (Kinsell, 1986)

D 100-500 mg/day PO (Kinsell, 1986)
25-75 mg IM, IV, SC (Kinsell, 1986)
100-500 mg PO q8h as urinary acidifier (Kinsell, 1986)

Gp 50 mg/day PO or parenterally (Williams, 1976)
200 mg/L in drinking water (Harkness and Wagner, 1977)
10mg/kg BW IM followed by oral supplementation (Bauck,1989)

Re Toroises: 10-20 mg/kg BW IM sid (Page and Mautino,1990)

Vitamin D_3

D 1-2 rounded tsp/10 lb BW PO sid, mix with feed or water (as a drench) (Kinsell, 1986)

N 2000 IU/kg BW in diet (Whitney et al, 1973)

Re 7,500 IU every 2 weeks IM (Snipes, 1984)
Tortoises: 1650 IU/kg BW IM once (Page and Mautino,1990)

Vitamin K_1

Bi 10-20 mg/kg BW IM sid, bid (Nemetz, 1990)
0.2-2.5 mg/kg BW IM for 1-2 injections (Harrison and Harrison, 1986)

Winstrol-V (stanozolol)

Bi 0.5-1 mg/kg BW IM (Harrison and Harrison, 1986)
2 mg/4 oz water [tablet form] (Nemetz, 1990)

C 10-25 mg IM weekly (Kinsell, 1986)

D 10-50 mg IM weekly (Kinsell, 1986)

Yohimbine

Ch 2.1 mg/kg BW IP (Hargett et al, 1989)

Go 0.2 mg/kg BW IV slowly over 1 minute (NCSU, 1987)

Gp 1.0 mg/kg BW IP (Strother and Stokes, 1989)

R   2.1 mg/kg BW IP (Hsu et al, 1986)

Rb 0.2 mg/kg BW IV (Keller et al, 1988)

Sh 0.2 mg/kg BW IV slowly over 1 minute (NCSU, 1987)

APPENDIXES

Table A.1. Bleeding sites

Bird
1) Brachial vein*
2) Cutaneous ulnar vein (NAS, 1977)
3) Right jugular vein (NAS, 1977)
4) Cardiac puncture#
5) Toe nail (Nemetz, 1990)
6) Medial metatarsal vein (NAS, 1977)

Cat
1) Cephalic vein*
2) Jugular vein*

Dog
1) Cephalic vein*
2) Jugular vein*

Ferret
1) Cephalic vein
2) Retro-orbital sinus#
3) Tail artery
4) Tarsal vein
5) Cardiac puncture#
6) Jugular vein*

Gerbil
1) Lateral tail vein
2) Retro-orbital plexus#
3) Cardiac puncture#
4) Abdominal aorta#
5) Tail tip amputation#

Guinea pig
1) Middle ear vein
2) Metatarsal vein
3) Cardiac puncture*#
4) Jugular vein (for exsanguination)#

Hamster
1) Retro-orbital plexus#
2) Jugular vein
3) Cardiac puncture#
4) Tail vein
5) Femoral vein

Mouse
1) Tail veins
2) Carotid artery
3) Retro-orbital plexus
4) Jugular vein
5) Cardiac puncture
6) Ear vein
7) Tail tip amputation*#

Non-human primates
1) Femoral vein*
2) Tail vein
3) Jugular vein
4) Saphenous vein
5) Cephalic vein*

Table A.1.   Bleeding sites (*continued*)

Pig
    1) Ear vein (nick or puncture)   3) Cranial vena cava*
    2) External jugular vein   4) Brachiocephalic vein

Rabbit
    1) Marginal ear vein*   3) Retro-orbital plexus#
    2) Cardiac puncture#   Not recommended by some
                                authors

Rat
    1) Tail veins*   3) Retro-orbital plexus#
    2) Sublingual vein   4) Cardiac puncture#
                                Not recommended by some
                                authors

*Preferred site
#Requires anesthesia or analgesia
Source: Adapted from *UFAW Handbook,* 1986, and Joint Working Group, 1993.

Table A.2.   Plasma and blood volume

Species	Plasma volume mean (range)	Blood volume mean (range)
	ml/kg	*ml/kg*
Cat	41 (35-52)	55 (47-66)
Cattle	38.8 (36.3-40.6)	57 (52-61)
Chicken	——	60
Dog	50.0	86 (79-90)
European Rabbit	39 (28-51)	56 (44-70)
Ferret	——	75
Frog	80	95
Gerbil	——	67
Goat	56	70 (57-89)
Guinea pig	39 (35-48)	75 (67-92)
Hamster	——	78
Marmot	51	100
Mouse	——	79
Opossum	38 (30-52)	57 (45-70)
Pig	——	65 (61-68)
Rat	40 (36-45)	64 (58-70)
Rhesus macaque	36 (30-48)	54 (44-67)
Sheep	47 (44-45)	66 (60-74)

Source: Adapted from Altman and Dittmer, 1974, and Joint Working Group, 1993.

Species	Body weight	Tube diameter	Laryngoscope
Canine	0.5-5 kg	2-5 mm O/D	MacIntosh size 1-4
	5 kg	4-15 mm O/D	
Feline	0.5-1.5 kg	2-3 mm O/D	MacIntosh size 1
	> 1.5 kg	3-4.5 mm O/D	
Gerbil	70-120 g	Not reported	
Goat	10-90 kg	5-15 mm O/D	MacIntosh size 2-4
Guinea pig	400-1000 g	1.5-2.5 mm O/D	
Hamster	70-120 g	Not reported	
Mouse	25-35 g		
Pig	1-10 kg	2-6 mm O/D	Soper or Wisconsin size 1-4
	10-200 kg	6-15 mm O/D	
Primate	0.5 kg	Not reported	MacIntosh size 1-3
	0.5-20 kg	2-8 mm O/D	
Rabbit	1-3 kg	2-3 mm O/D	Wisconsin size 0-1
	3-7 kg	3-6 mm O/D	
Rat	200-400 g	16-21 gauge plastic cannula	
Sheep	10-90 kg	5-15 mm O/D	MacIntosh size 2-4
Bird	<500 g	8-12 French feeding tube	
	>500 g	4-6 mm O/D (non-cuffed)	

Source: From Flecknell, 1987; except 'Bird' from Nemetz, 1990 (reprinted by permission).

Table A.4. Needle sizes, sites, and recommended volumes for injection

Species	SC	IM	IP	IV
			Injection Site	
Feline	Scruff, back, 50-100 ml, <20G	Quadriceps/caudal thigh, 1 ml, <20G	50-100 ml, <20G	Cephalic vein, 2-5 ml (slowly), <21G
Canine	Scruff, back, 100-200 ml, <20G	Quadriceps/caudal thigh, 2-5 ml, <20G	200-500 ml, <20G	Cephalic vein, 10-15 ml (slowly), <20G
Ferret	Scruff, 20-30 ml, <20G	Quadriceps/caudal thigh, 0.5-1 ml, <20G	50-100 ml, <20G	Cephalic vein, 2-5 ml (slowly), <21G
Guinea pig	Scruff, back, 5-10 ml, <20G	Quadriceps/caudal thigh, 0.3 ml, <21G	10-15 ml, <21G 0.5 ml, <23G	Ear vein, saphenous vein
Hamster	Scruff, 3-4 ml, <20G	Quadriceps/caudal thigh, 0.1 ml, <21G	3-4 ml, <21G	Femoral or jugular vein (cut down), 0.3 ml, <25G
Mouse	Scruff, 2-3 ml, <20G	Quadriceps/caudal thigh, 0.05 ml, <23G	2-3 ml, <21G	Lateral tail vein, 0.2 ml, <25G
Primate (Marmoset)	Scruff, 5-10 ml, <20G	Quadriceps/caudal thigh, 0.3-0.5 ml, <21G	10-15 ml, <21G	Lateral tail vein, 0.5-1 ml (slowly), <21G

Primate (Baboon)	Scruff, 10-30 ml, <20G	Quadriceps/caudal thigh, triceps, 1-3 ml, <20G	50-100 ml, <20G	Cephalic vein, recurrent tarsal vein, jugular vein, 10-20 ml (slowly), <20G
Rabbit	Scruff, flank, 30-50 ml, <20G	Quadriceps/caudal thigh, lumbar muscles 0.5-1.0 ml, 20G	50-100 ml, <20G	Marginal ear vein, 1-5 ml (slowly), <21G
Rat	Scruff, 5-10 ml, <20G	Quadriceps/caudal thigh, 0.3 ml, <21G	5-10 ml, <21G	Lateral tail vein, 0.5 ml, <23G
Bird	Pectoral, interscapular, or inguinal fold 1-3% BW bid or tid <21G	Pectoral/per site 0.2 ml/<100 g BW 0.2-0.5 ml/100-500 g BW 0.5-1.0 ml/>500 g BW <25G	Not applicable	Cutaneous ulnar vein <25G short bevel

Source: From Flecknell, 1987; except 'Bird' from Nemetz, 1990 (reprinted by permission).

Table A.5. Body surface area conversions

kg	M²	kg	M²
0.5	0.06	26.0	0.88
1.0	0.10	27.0	0.90
2.0	0.15	28.0	0.92
3.0	0.20	29.0	0.94
4.0	0.25	30.0	0.96
5.0	0.29	31.0	0.99
6.0	0.33	32.0	1.01
7.0	0.36	33.0	1.03
8.0	0.40	34.0	1.05
9.0	0.43	35.0	1.07
10.0	0.46	36.0	1.09
11.0	0.49	37.0	1.11
12.0	0.52	38.0	1.13
13.0	0.55	39.0	1.15
14.0	0.58	40.0	1.17
15.0	0.60	41.0	1.19
16.0	0.63	42.0	1.21
17.0	0.66	43.0	1.23
18.0	0.69	44.0	1.25
19.0	0.71	45.0	1.26
20.0	0.74	46.0	1.28
21.0	0.76	47.0	1.30
22.0	0.78	48.0	1.32
23.0	0.81	49.0	1.34
24.0	0.83	50.0	1.36
25.0	0.85		

Note: M^2 = weight $(g)^{2/3} \times K \times 10^{-4}$; where K = 10.1 for cats and dogs; 10.5 for mice. M = meters.

Table A.6. Safe bleeding volume

Species	One bleeding (maximium)	Species	One bleeding (maximum)
	ml/kg		*ml/kg*
Cat	7.7	Horse	8.8
Cattle	7.7	Monkey (Macaque)	6.6
Chicken	9.9	Mouse	7.7
Dog	9.9	Pig	6.6
Goat	6.6	Rabbit	7.7
Guinea Pig	7.7	Rat	5.5
Hamster	5.5	Sheep	6.6

Source: Adapted from Mitruka and Rawnsley, 1977.

Table A.7. Toxic doses of antibiotics in rodents

Antibiotic	Mouse	Rat	Guinea pig	Hamster
Penicillin			5000 IU IP: 60% mortality 10000 IU PO: 20% mortality 1000000 IU IM, two doses in 24 hours: ⅞ died	100 mg PO, 600 mg SC: 100% mortality within 5 days
Procaine	0.3 mg/kg: 90% mortality		0.4 mg/kg, 125 mg/kg: 100% with convulsions	
Ampicillin			8 mg/kg SC tid for 5 days: 20% mortality by day 8	5 mg PO tid 5 days: 90% mortality
Cephalosporins			Cefazolin, 100 mg IM qid 5 days: ³⁄₂ died	Cephalexin, 5 mg PO tid 5 days: 90% mortality Cefoxitin 10 mg IM tid 5 days: 100% motality Cephalothin 20 mg IM tid 5 days: 80% mortality
Carbenicillin				100 mg/kg PO: ⁹⁄₁₀ animals died within 8 days
Ticarcillin				100 mg/kg PO: ¹⁰⁄₁₀ animals died within 6 days
Lincomycin			30 mg/kg SC on alternate days: most animals died 5-14 days after treatment started	>10 mg/kg SC: ²³⁄₂₄ animals died with enteritis
Clindamycin			75 mg/kg IP sid: 100% mortality in 6-8 days	3 mg PO tid 5 days: 100% mortality
Streptomycin	6 mg/kg IM:		60 mg per animal once PO:	Acutely lethal at *therapeutic* dose rates

Drug				
Neomycin				285 mg/kg PO: death within 5 days
Chloramphenicol				10 mg PO tid for 5 days: 20% mortality; ≥300 mg/kg PO: enteritis
Erythromycin			Oral ≥ 33 mg/kg for 3 days: 40% mortality; 33 mg/kg IP: 100% mortality	5 mg PO tid 5 days: 100% mortality; 30-200 mg/lg IP: 100% mortality
Aureomycin			5 mg/kg PO: 100% mortality; 100 μg/kg in diet: % died	
Tetracycline	150 mg/kg		50 mg/kg in diet	100 mg/kg PO: majority of animals died within 3-4 days
Chlortetracycline			20 mg/animal PO: mortality % not given	
Vancomycin				5 mg PO tid 5 days: 90% mortality
Bacitracin			2000 IU/animal: 80% mortality	
Spiramycin	3.13 g/kg: acute oral LD$_{50}$	4.85 g/kg: acute oral LD$_{50}$	3.5 g/kg: acute oral LD$_{50}$; 0.25 g/kg: chronic oral LD$_{50}$ with enteritis	
Trimethoprim-sulfamethoxazole				33 mg trimethoprim, 167 mg sulfamethoxazole/kg PO: ‰ animals died

Source: Morris, 1995, (reprinted by permission). See Morris, 1995, for references.

Table A.8.   Adverse effects of antibiotic treatment in rabbits

Antiobiotic	Toxic dose	Toxic effects
Ampicillin	25 mg/kg IM for 2 days	Fatal enteritin
	5 mg/kg IM for 2 days	Weight loss
	40 mg/kg SC for 4 days	40% fatal enteritis over next 2 weeks
	10 mg/kg PO for 6 days	50% fatal enteritis over next month
	8 mg/kg bid SC	Enteritis, previously also had penicillin
	> 5mg/kg PO antibiotic treated water for 3 days	Fatal enteritin in 7/11 rabbits
Penicillin	LD$_{50}$ 5.25 g/kg PO	Both acute and chronic toxicity (enteritis)
Cephalexin	200 mg/rabbit for 7 days	Diarrhea
Lincomycin	100 mg PO single dose in 1.5-2.0 kg rabbits	66% mortality with enteritis
	24 mg/kg PO antibiotic treated water	90 % mortality with enteritis
	30 mg/day PO in 2.0-2.5 kn rabbits	100% mortality with enteritis by 3 days
	1.3 mg/adult rabbit in feed for 3 days	$^{20}/_{30}$ rabbits died with enteritis
	0.2 mg/kg IM for 2 days	33% mortality in 2 days
Clindamycin	15 mg/kg PO for 3 days	100% mortality with enteritis
	5 mg/kg PO for 2 days	50% mortality with enteritis within 72 hours
	Single IV dose of 30 mg/kg	⅘ rabbits had fatal enteritis 12-14 days after treatment
Tylosin	100 mg/rabbit for 7 days	Diarrhea
Erythromycin	3 g/L in drinking water for 7 days	Diarrhea
Spectinomycin	1 g/L in drinking water for 7 days	Diarrhea
Vancomycin	75 mg/kg IV	Acute toxicity with 100% mortality
Minocycline	30 mg/kg IM for 3 days	Reduction in growth rate
Spiramycin	Acute oral LD$_{50}$ 4.85 g/kg	Nervous signs

REFERENCES

Adam, H.K., J.B. Glen, and P.A. Hoyle. Pharmacokinetics in laboratory animals of ICI 35868, a new I.V. anesthetic agent. Br. J. Anaesth. 52: 743-746, 1990.

Albengres, E., J.L. Pinquier, P. Riant, F. Bree, S. Urien, J. Barre, and J.P. Tillement. Pharmacological criterion for risk-benefit evaluation of NSAIDS. Scand. J. Rheumatol. Suppl. 73: 3-15, 1988.

Alder, V.A., D. Yu, E. Su, and S.J. Cringle. Comparison of hematologic parameters in normal and streptozotocin-induced diabetic rats. Lab. Anim. Sci. 42:170-173, 1992.

Altman, P.L. and D.S. Dittmer. *The Biology Data Book,* 2nd ed Federation of the American Society of Experimental Biologists, Bethesda, MD, 1974.

Andrews, P.L.R., and O. Illman. The ferret. In: *UFAW Handbook on the Care and Management of Laboratory Animals,* 6th ed. T. Poole, ed. Churchill Livingstone Inc., New York, 1987.

Balazs, T., A.M. Hatch, E.R.W. Gregory, and H.C. Grice. A comparative study of hymenolpicides in *Hymenolepis nana* infestation of rats. Can. J. Comp. Med. Vet. Sci. 26: 160-162, 1962.

Balser, D.S. Tranquilizer tabs for capturing wild carnivores. J. Wildl. Manage. 29(3): 438-442, 1965.

Banerjee, A.K., A.F. Angulo, K.M. Dhasmana, and J. Kon-A-San. Acute diarrhoeal disease in rabbit: Bacteriological diagnosis and efficacy of oral rehydration in combination with loperamide hydrochloride. Lab. Anim. 21: 314-317, 1987.

Barthold, S.W. The microbiology of transmissible murine colonic hyperplasia. Lab. Anim. Sci. 30(2): 167-173, 1980.

Bartlett, J.G. Antibiotic associated pseudomembranous colitis. Rev. Infect. Dis. 1: 530-539, 1979.

Bartlett, J.G., T. Chang, N. Moon, and A.B. Onderdonk. Antibiotic-induced lethal enterocolitis in hamsters: Studies with eleven agents and evidence to support the pathogenic role of toxin-producing clostridia. Am. J. Vet. Res. 39(9): 1525-1530, 1978.

Battles, A.H., S.W. Adams, C.H. Courtney, and C.R.T. Mladinich. Efficacy of ivermectin against natural infection of *Syphacia muris* in rats. Lab. Anim. Sci. 37(6): 791-792, 1987.

Battles, A.H., E.C. Greiner, and B.R. Collins. Efficacy of ivermectin against natural infection of *Strongyloides* spp. in squirrel monkeys (*Saimiri sciureus*). Lab. Anim. Sci. 38(4): 474-476, 1988.

Bauck, L. Ophthalmic conditions in pet rabbits and rodents. Compend. Contin. Educ. Pract. Vet. 11(3): 258-268, 1989.

Bayer, A.S., D. Norman, and D. Anderson. Efficacy of ciprofloxacin in experimental arthritis caused by *Escherichia coli*—in vitro-in vivo correlations. J. Infect. Dis. 152(4): 811-816, 1985.

Bell, G.R. A guide to the properties, characteristics, and uses of some general anesthetics for fish. Bull. Fish. Res. Board Can. 148, 1964.

Bell, J.A. Parasites of domesticated pet ferrets. Compend. Contin. Educ. Pract. Vet. 16:617-620, 1994.

Ben, M., R.L. Dixon, and R.H. Adamson. Anesthesia in the rat. Fed. Proc. 28:1522-1527, 1969.

Blair, L.S., and P.E. Thompson. Effects of pyrvinium pamoate in the ration or drinking water of rats against the pinworm *Syphacia muris*. Lab. Anim. Care 19(5): 639-643, 1969.

Blake, D.W., B. Jover, and B.P. McGrath. Haemodynamic and heart rate reflex responses to propofol in the rabbit. Br. J. Anaesth. 61: 194-199, 1988.

Boothe, D.M. Drug therapy in cats: Recommended dosing regimens. J. Am. Vet. Med. Assoc. 196(11): 1845-1850, 1990.

Borchard, R.E., C.D. Barnes, and L.G. Eltherington. *Drug Dosage in Laboratory Animals: A Handbook,* 3rd ed. The Telford Press, Inc, Caldwell, NJ, 1990.

Boss, S.M., C.L. Gries, B.K. Kirchner, G.D. Smith, and P.C. Francis. Use of vancomycin hydrochloride for treatment of *Clostridium difficile* enteritis in Syrian hamsters. Lab. Anim. Sci. 44: 31-37, 1994.

Bowman, T.A., and J.W. Griffith. Comparison of treatments for *Psorergates* mites in stumptailed macaques (*Macaca arctoides*). Lab. Anim. Sci. 37(1): 100-102, 1987.

Brooks, D.L. Coccidiosis and other rabbit parasites. Rabbit Health Symposium, Fort Collins, CO, 1(1), 1979.

Broome, R.L., D.L. Brooks, J.G. Babish, D.D. Copeland, and G.M. Conzelman. Pharmacokinetic properties of enroflosacin in rabbits. Am J. Vet. Res. 52:1835-1841, 1991.

Burk, T.J. Rats, mice, hamsters, and gerbils. Small Anim. Pract. 9(3): 473-486, 1979.

Burk, T.J. Antibiotic therapy in pet birds and reptiles. In: *Veterinary Pharmaceuticals and Biologicals.* Veterinary Medicine Publishing Co., Lenexa, KA, 1986.

Bush, M., R.S. Custer, J.M. Smeller, and P. Charache. Recommendations for antibiotic therapy in reptiles. In: *Reproductive Biology and Diseases of Captive Reptiles.* J.B. Murphy and J.T Collins, eds., 223-226. Meseraull Printing, Lawrence, KA, 1980.

Carter, K.K., S.H. Hietala, D.L. Brooks, and J.D. Baggot. Tylosin concentrations in rat serum and lung tissue after administration in drinking water. Lab. Anim. Sci. 37(4): 468-470, 1987.

CCAC (Canadian Council on Animal Care). *Guide to the Care and Use of Experimental Animals,* vols. I and II. Canadian Council on Animal Care, Ontario, Canada, 1984.

Clifford, D.R. What the practicing veterinarian should know about gerbils. VM/SAC 68(8): 912-918, 1973.

Clifford, D.H. Preanesthesia, anesthesia, analgesia, and euthanasia. In: *Laboratory Animal Medicine,* J.G. Fox et al., eds., 527-562. ACLAM Laboratory Animal Medicine Series. Academic Press, New York, 1984.

Coghlan, L.G., D.R. Lee, B. Psencik, and D. Weiss. Practical and effective eradication of pinworms (*Syphacia muris*) in rats by use of fenbendazole. Lab. Anim. Sci. 43:481-487, 1993.

Cooper, J. Amphibians. In: *Manual of Exotic Pets.* Cooper et al, eds. British Small Animal Veterinary Association, Cheltenham, UK, 1985.

Cooper, J.E. Anaesthesia of exotic animals. Anim. Tech. 35(1): 13-20, 1984.

Cox, A.K., D.W. Morck, and M.E. Olson. Evaluation of detomidine and ketamine-detomidine for anesthesia in laboratory rats. Contemp. Top. Lab. Anim. Sci. 33: 52-55, 1994.

Cramlet, S.H., and E.F. Jones. Selected topics in laboratory animal medicine. 5. Anesthesiology. USAF School of aerospace medicine, Brooks Air Force Base, Texas, 1976.

Crawshaw, G.J. Amphibian medicine. In: *Zoo & Wild Animal Medicine. Current Therapy 3.* M.E. Fowler, ed., 131-139. W.B. Saunders Company, Philadelphia, 1993.

Croft, P.G. *An Introduction to the Anaesthesia of Laboratory Animals.* UFAW, London, 1964.

Cummins, L.B., M.E. Keeling, and H.M. McClure. Preventive medicine in anthropoids: Parasite control. Lab. Anim. Sci. 23(5): 819-822, 1973.

Cunliffe-Beamer, T.L, and R.R. Fox. Venereal spirochetosis of rabbits: Eradication. Lab. Anim. Sci. 31(4): 379-381, 1981.

Curl, J.L., J.S. Curl, and J.K. Harrison. Pharmacokinetics of long acting oxytetracycline in the laboratory rat. Lab. Anim. Sci. 38(4): 430-434, 1988.

DaRif, C.A., and H.G. Rush. Management of septicemia in rhesus monkeys with chronic indwelling venous catheters. Lab. Anim. Sci. 33(1): 90-94, 1983.

Deeb, B.J., P. Eyman, M.L. Hutton, and L.C. Abbott. Efficacy of synthetic opioid analgesics administered in drinking water of rats. Lab. Anim. Sci. 39(5): 473, 1989 (Abstract).

Delbarre, B., and G. Delbarre. Effect of indapamide on an experimental model of cerebral ischemia in hypertensive rats. Am. J. Med. 84(1B): 20-25, 1988.

Dixon, L.W. Antibiotic toxicosis in the guinea pig. Texas Vet. Med. J. 48:31, 1986.

Doerning, B.J., D.W. Brammer, C.E. Chrisp, and H.G. Rush. Anesthetic and nephrotoxic effects of Tiletamine/Zolazepam in rabbits. Lab. Anim. Sci. 40(5): 562, 1990 (Abstract).

Doerning, B.J., D.W. Brammer, C.E. Chrisp, and H.G. Rush. Nephrotoxicity of tiletamine in New Zealand White rabbits. Lab. Anim. Sci. 42:267-269, 1992.

Dolowy, W.C., P. Mombelloni, and A.L. Hesse. Chlorpromazine premedication with pentobarbital anesthesia in a mouse. Am. J. Vet. Res. 21: 156-157, 1960.

Domino, E.F., D.A. McCarthy, and G.A. Deneau. General anesthesia in infrahuman primates. Fed. Proc. 28(4): 1500-1509, 1969.

Dorrestein, G.M. Enrofloxacin in pet avian and exotic animal therapy. In: *Proceedings of the 1st International Baytril Symposium.* A.G. Bayer, ed., 63-70. Bonn, Germany, 1992.

Duwel, D., and K. Brech. Control of oxyuriasis in rabbits by fenbendazole. Lab. Anim. 15: 101-105, 1981.

Eberhard, M.L. Chemotherapy of filariasis in squirrel monkeys (*Saimiri sciureus*). Lab. Anim. Sci. 32(4): 397-400, 1982.

Egerton, J.R., J. Birnbaum, L.S. Blair, J.C. Chabala, J. Conroy, M.H. Fisher, H. Mrozik, D.A. Ostlind, C.A. Wilkins, and W.C. Campbell. 22-23-dihydroavermectin B-1, a new broad-spectrum antiparasitic agent. Br. Vet. J. 136: 88-97, 1980.

Ellison D.H., H. Velazquez, and F.S. Wright. Thiazide-sensitive sodium chloride cotransport in early distal tubule. Am. J. Physiol. 253: F546-F554, 1987.

Evans, A.T., and R.H. Evans. Raising raccoons for release. Part 4. Medical management and readiness for the wild. Vet. Tech. 7(1): 37-48, 1986.

Farrar, W.E., Jr., and T.H. Kent Enteritis and coliform bacteremia in guinea pigs given penicillin. Am. J. Pathol. 47(4): 629-642, 1965.

Farris, H.E., Jr. Office of University Research, Clemson University. Personal communication, January, 1990.

Feeser, P., and F. White. Medical management of *Lemur catta, Varecia varegata*, and *Propithecus verreauxi* in natural habitat enclosures. In: *Proceedings of the Annual Meeting of the American Association of Zoo Veterinarians,* Oakland, CA, 1992, pp. 320-323.

Findon, G., and T.E. Miller. Treatment of *Trichosomoides crassicauda* in laboratory rats using ivermectin. Lab. Anim. Sci. 37(4): 496-499, 1987.

Fineg, J., W.C. Hanly, J.R. Prine, D.C. Van Riper, and P.W. Day. Isoniazid therapy in the chimpanzee. Lab. Anim. Care 16: 436-446, 1966.

Finegold, M.J., M.E. Seaquist, and M.J. Doherty. Treatment of pulmonary acariasis in rhesus monkeys with an organic phosphate. Lab. Anim. Care 18(2): 127-130, 1968.

Flatt, R.E., S.H. Weisbroth, and A.L. Kraus. Metabolic, traumatic, mycotic, and miscellaneous diseases of rabbits. In: *The Biology of the Laboratory Rabbit.* S.H. Weisbroth. R.E. Flatt, and A.L. Krauss, eds., 435-451. Academic Press, New York, 1974

Flecknell, P.A. The management of post-operative pain and distress in experimental animals. Anim. Tech. 36(2): 97-103, 1985.

Flecknell, P.A. *Laboratory Animal Anesthesia.* Academic Press, London, Engl., 1987.

Flecknell, P.A. Presented at the American Association for Laboratory Animal Science Annual Meeting, Little Rock, AR, 1989.

Flecknell, P.A. Post-operative analgesia in rabbits and rodents. Lab. Anim. 20(9):34-37, 1991.

Forsythe, D.B., A.J. Payton, D. Dixon, P.H. Myers, J.A. Clark, and J.R. Snipe. Evaluation of Telazol-xylazine as an anesthetic combination for use in Syrian hamsters. Lab. Anim. Sci. 42:497-502, 1992.

Fowler, M.E. *Restraint and Handling of Wild and Domestic Animals.* Iowa State University Press, Ames, 1978.

Fraser, C.M., ed. Management, husbandry, diseases of laboratory animals: Diseases of nonhuman primates. In: *The Merck Veterinary Manual*, 7th ed, 1032-1036. Rahway, NJ, Merck & Co, 1991.

French, A.W. Elimination of *Ornithonyssus bacoti* in a colony of aging mice. Lab. Anim. Sci. 37(5): 670-672, 1987.

Fritz, D.E., W.J. Hurst, W.J. White, C.M. Lang. Pharmacokinetics of cefazolin in guinea pigs. Lab. Anim. Sci. 37:646-651, 1987.

Fromtling, R.A., G.K. Abruzzo, E.C. Gilfillan, B.A. Pelak, and H.H. Gadebusch. Norfloxacin versus trimethoprim-sulphamethoxazole: Efficacy in a model of ascending urinary tract infection in normal and streptozotocin-induced diabetic mice. J. Antimicrob. Chemother. 16(6): 735-741, 1985.

Frost, W.W. *Prevention and Control of Laboratory Animal Disease: A Therapeutic and Prophylactic Compendium*. ACLAM Laboratory Animal Medicine and Science Series. G.L. Van Hoosier, coord., University of Washington, Seattle, WA, 1977.

Frye, F.L. *Biomedical and Surgical Aspects of Captive Reptile Husbandry.* Veterinary Medicine Publ., Edwardsville, KA, 981.

Goelz, M., J. Thigpen, J. Mahler, W. Rogers, J. Locklear, B. Weigler, and D. Forsythe. The efficacy of various therapeutic regimens in eliminating *Pasteurella pneumotropica* from the mouse. Contemp. Top. Lab. Anim. Sci. 33: A-3, 1994 (Abstract). Note: Misprint of dose reported by author, personal communication. Correct dose is listed.

Grad, R., M.L. Witten, S.F. Quan, D.H. McKelvie, and R.J. Lemen. Intravenous chloralose is a safe anesthetic for longitudinal use in beagle puppies. Lab. Anim. Sci. 38(4): 422-425, 1988.

Green, C.J. *Animal Anesthesia: Laboratory Animal Handbooks 8, Laboratory Animals.* LTD, London, 1982.

Green, C.J., J. Knight, S. Precious, et al. Metomidate, etomidate and fentanyl as injectable anesthetic agents in mice. Lab. Anim. 15:171-175, 1981.

Guide to care and use of nudes. ILAR News. 19(2), 1976.

Habermann, R.T., and F.P. Williams. The efficacy of some piperazine compounds and stylomycin in drinking water for the removal of oxyurids from mice and rats and a method of critical testing of anthelmintics. Proc. Anim. Care Panel 7(2): 89-97, 1957.

Hargett, C.E., Jr., J.W. Record, M. Carrier, Jr., K.C. Bordwell, and J.H. Patterson, Jr. Reversal of ketamine-xylazine anesthesia in the chinchilla by yohimbine. Lab. Anim. 18(7): 41-43, 1989.

Harkness, J.E., and J.E. Wagner. *The Biology and Medicine of Rabbits and Rodents.* Lea and Febiger, Philadelphia, PA, 1977.

Harkness, J.E., and J.E. Wagner. *The Biology and Medicine of Rabbits and Rodents,* 2nd ed. Lea and Febiger, Philadelphia, PA, 1983.

Harkness, J.E., and J.E. Wagner. *The Biology and Medicine of Rabbits and Rodents,* 3rd ed. Lea and Febiger, Philadelphia, PA, 1989.

Harrison, G.J., and L.R. Harrison. *Clinical Avian Medicine and Surgery.* W.B. Saunders Co., Philadelphia, 1986.

Haskins, S.C. Use of analgesics postoperatively and in a small animal intensive care setting. J. Am. Vet. Med. Assoc. 191(10): 1266-1268, 1987.

Hatch, R.C. The effect of glucose, sodium lactate, and epinephrine on thiopental anesthesia in dogs. J. Am. Vet. Med. Assoc. 148: 135-140, 1966.

Heaton, J.T., and S.E. Brauth. Effects of yohimbine as a reversing agent for ketamine-xylazine anesthesia in budgerigars. Lab. Anim. Sci. 42:54-56, 1992.

Hoag, W.G. Oxyuriasis in laboratory mouse colonies. Am. J. Vet. Res. 22: 150-153, 1961.

Hofing, G.L. Guidelines for the use of analgesics, anesthetics, and tranquilizers. Parke-Davis Corp., 1989.

Holmes, D.D. *Clinical Laboratory Animal Medicine.* Iowa State University Press, Ames, 1984.

Hrapkiewicz, K.L., S. Stein, and K.L. Smiler. A new anesthetic agent for use in the gerbil. Lab. Anim. Sci. 39(4): 338-341, 1989.

Hsu, C.K. Parasitic diseases, In: *The Laboratory Rat,* vol. 1. H.J. Baker, J.R. Lindsey, and S.H. Weisbroth, eds., 307-331. Academic Press, New York, 1979.

Hsu, W.H., S.I. Bellin, H.D. Dellmann, and C.E. Hanson. Xylazine-ketamine-induced anesthesia in rats and its antagonism by yohimbine. J. Am. Vet. Med. Assoc. 189(9): 1040, 1986.

Huerkamp, M.J. Letter. Lab. Anim. Sci. 40(1): 5, 1990.

Huerkamp, M.J. Ivermectin eradication of pinworms from rats kept in ventilated cages. Lab. Anim. Sci. 43:86-90, 1993.

Hughes, H.C. Anesthesia of laboratory animals. Lab. Anim. 10(5): 40-56, 1981.

Hughes, H.C., W.J. White, and C.M. Lang. Guidelines for the use of tranquilizers, anesthetics, and analgesics in laboratory animals. Vet. Anesth. 2: 19-24, 1975.

Ialeggio, D.M. Practical medicine of primate pets. Compend. Contin. Educ. Pract. Vet. 11(10): 1252-1258, 1989.

Isaza, R., B. Baker, and F. Dunker. Medical management of inflammatory bowel disease in a spider monkey. J. Am. Vet. Med. Assoc. 200: 1543, 1992.

Jackson Laboratory, The. Animal Resources, Bar Harbor, ME.

Jacobson, E.R. Diseases of reptiles, Part 2: Infectious diseases. Compend. Contin. Educ. Pract. Vet. 3: 195-199, 1981.

Jaslow, B.W., D.H. Ringler, H.G. Rush, and J.C. Glorioso. *Pasteurella* associated rhinitis of rabbits: Efficacy of penicillin therapy. Lab. Anim. Sci. 31(4): 382-385, 1981.

Jenkins, W.L. Pharmacologic aspects of analgesic drugs in animals: An overview. J. Am. Vet. Med. Assoc. 191(10): 1231-140, 1987.

Johnson, D.K., R.J. Russell, and J.A. Stunkard. *A Guide to Diagnosis, Treatment, and Husbandry of Nonhuman Primates.* Veterinary Medicine Publ., Edwardsville, KA, 1981.

Joint Working Group on Refinements. Removal of blood from laboratory animals and birds. Lab. Anim. 27:1-22, 1993.

Junge, R.E., K.G. Mehren, et al. Hypertrophic osteoarthropathy and renal disease in three black lemurs (*Lemur macaco*). In: *Proceedings of the Annual Meeting of the American Association of Zoo Veterinarians,* Oakland, CA, 320-323, 1992.

Kaplan, H.M. Anesthesia in amphibians and reptiles. Fed. Proc. 28: 1541-1546, 1969.

Kapusnik, J.E., C.J. Hackbarth, H.F. Chambers, T. Carpenter, and M.A. Sande. Single, large, daily dosing versus intermittent dosing of tobramycin for treating experimental pseudomonas pneumonia. J. Infect. Dis. 158(1): 7-12, 1988.

Keller, G.L., D.H. Bauman, and L. Abbott. Yohimbine antagonism of ketamine and xylazine anesthesia in rabbits. Lab. Anim. 17(3): 28-30, 1988.

Kelly, D.J., J.D. Chulary, et al. Serum concentrations of penicillin, doxycycline, and ciprofloxacin during prolonged therapy in rhesus monkeys. J. Infect. Dis. 166:1184-1187, 1992.

Kinsell, R., Ed. *Formulary.* Purdue University School of Veterinary Medicine Pharmacy, 1986.

Klontz, G.W. Anesthesia in fishes. In: *Anesthesia in Experimental Animals.* (Proceedings of a symposium) Brooks Air Force Base, Texas, 1964.

Ko, J.C.H., J.C. Thurmon, W.J. Tranquilli, G.J. Benson, and W.A. Olson. A comparison of medetomidine-propofol and medetomidine-midazolam-propofol anesthesia in rabbits. Lab. Anim. Sci. 42:503-507, 1992.

Ko, J.C.H., B.L. Williams, V.L. Smith, C.J. McGrath, and J.D. Jacobson. Comparison of Telazol, Telazol-ketamine, Telazol-xylazine, and Telazol-ketamine-xylazine as chemical restraint and anesthetic induction combination in swine. Lab. Anim. Sci. 43:476-480, 1993.

Krueger, K.L., J.C. Murphy, and J.G. Fox. Treatment of proliferative colitis in ferrets. J. Am. Vet. Med. Assoc. 194(10): 1435-1436, 1989.

La Regina, M., W.H. Fales, and J.E. Wagner Effects of antibiotic treatment on the occurrence of experimentally induced proliferative ileitis of hamsters. Lab. Anim. Sci. 30(1): 38-41, 1980.

Lawrence, K., P.W. Muggleton, and J.R. Needham. Preliminary study on the use of ceftazidime, a broad spectrum cephalosporin antibiotic, in snakes. Res. Vet. Sci. 36:16-20, 1984.

Le Blanc, S.A., R.E. Faith, C.A. Montgomery. Use of topical ivermectin treatment for *Syphacia obvelata* in mice. Lab. Anim. Sci. 43:526-538, 1993.

Letcher, J., and M. Glade. Efficacy of ivermectin as an anthelmintic in leopard frogs. J. Am. Vet. Med. Assoc. 200: 537-538, 1992.

Lewis, G.E., and P.B. Jennings, Jr. Effective sedation of laboratory animals using Innovar. Vet. Lab. Anim. Sci. 22(3): 430-432, 1972.

Liles, J.H., and P.A. Flecknell. The use of non-steroidal anti-inflammatory drugs for the relief of pain in laboratory rodents and rabbits. Lab. Anim. 26: 241-255, 1992.

Line, A.S. Comments on Baytril antimicrobial therapy and considerations for intramuscular antibiotic therapy in captive primates. Lab. Primate Newsl. 32:3, 1993.

Line, A.S., J. Paul-Murphy, D.P. Aucoin, and D.C. Hirsh. Enrofloxacin treatment of long-tailed macaques with acute bacillary dysentery due to multiresistant *Shigella flexneri* IV. Lab. Anim. Sci. 42:240-244, 1992.

Lipman, N.S., P.A. Phillips, and C.E. Newcomer. Reversal of ketamine/xylazine anesthesia in the rabbit with yohimbine. Lab. Anim. Sci. 37(4): 474-477, 1987.

Lipman, N.S., A.K. Weischedel, D.A. Olson, and M.J. Conway. Treatment modality for clindamycin induced enterocolitis in the rabbit. Lab. Anim. Sci. 39(5): 486, 1989 (Abstract).

Lumb, W.V., and E.W. Jones. *Veterinary Anesthesia,* 2nd ed. Lea & Febiger, Philadelphia, 1984.

Mann, D.R., D.C. Collins, M.M. Smith, M.J. Kessler, and K.G. Gould. Treatment of endometriosis in monkeys: Effectiveness of continuous infusion of a gonadotropin-releasing hormone agonist compared to treatment with a progestational steroid. J. Clin. Endocrinol. Metab. 63(6): 1277-1283, 1986.

Marangos, M.N., C.O. Onyeji, D.P. Nicolau, and C.H. Nightingale. Aspirin disposition in rabbits. Contemp. Top. Lab. Anim. Sci. 33: A-24, 1994 (Abstract).

Marcus, L.C. Bacterial infections in reptiles. In: *Reproductive Biology and Diseases of Captive Reptiles.* J.B. Murphy and J.T. Collins, eds., 211-221. Meseraull Printing, Lawrence, KA, 1980.

Marcus, L.C. *Veterinary Biology and Medicine of Captive Amphibians and Reptiles.* Lea and Febiger, Philadelphia, PA, 1981.

Marini, R.P., N.S. Lipman, and S. Erdman. A comparison of ketamine-xylazine and ketamine-xylazine-acepromazine anesthesia in the rabbit. Lab. Anim. Sci. 39(5): 482, 1989 (Abstract).

McDonald, S.E. Common anesthetic dosages for use in psittacine birds. J. Assoc. Avian Vet. 3(4): 186-187, 1989.

McDonald, S.E., and M.J. Lavoipierre. *Trixacarus caviae* infestation in two guinea pigs. Lab. Anim. Sci. 30: 67-70, 1980.

McDougall, P.T., N.S. Wolf, W.A. Stenback, and J.J. Trentin. Control of *Pseudomonas aeruginosa* in an experimental mouse colony. Lab. Anim. Care 17(2): 204-214, 1967.

McKellar, Q.A. Drug dosages for small mammals. Practice (March):57-61, 1989.

McKellar, Q.A., D.M. Midgley, E.A. Galbraith, E.W. Scott, and A. Bradley. Clinical and pharmacological properties of ivermectin in rabbits and guinea pigs. Vet. Rec. 130:71-73, 1992.

Melby, E.C., and N.H. Altman, eds. *CRC Handbook of Laboratory Animal Science,* vol. 3. CRC Press, Cleveland, OH, 1976.

Mitruka, B.M., and H.M. Rawnsley. *Clinical, Biochemical, and Hematological Reference Values in Normal Experimental Animals and Normal Humans.* Masson Publishing USA, Inc., New York, 1977.

Mladinich, C.R.J. Rabbits! "What's up, doc?" Vet. Forum (September): 28-30, 1989.

Moreland, A.F., and C. Glaser. Evaluation of ketamine, ketamine-xylazine and ketamine-diazepam anesthesia in the ferret. Lab. Anim. Sci. 35(3): 287-290, 1985.

Morris, T.M. Antibiotic therapeutics in laboratory animals. Lab. Anim. 29(1): 16-36, 1995.

Morton, D.B., and P.H.M Griffiths. Guidelines on the recognition of pain, distress and discomfort in experimental animals and an hypothesis for assessment. Vet. Rec. 116:431-436, 1985.

Murphy, J.B. The use of macrolide antibiotic tylosin in the treatment of reptilian respiratory infections. Br. J. Herpetol. 4: 317-321, 1973.

NAS. Laboratory Animal Management: Wild Birds. Committee on Birds, Institute of Laboratory Animal Resources, National Research Council, National Academy of Sciences, Washington, DC, 1977.

NCSU. North Carolina State University Section on Anesthesia, NC State University School of Veterinary Medicine, 1987.

Nemetz, L.P. Personal communication. The B.I.R.D. Clinic, Santa Ana, CA 92701.

Nicolau, D.P., C.D. Freeman, C.H. Nightingale, and R. Quintiliani. Pharmacokinetics of minocycline and vancomycin in rabbits. Lab. Anim. Sci. 43:222-225, 1993.

Norden, C.W., and E. Shinners. Ciprofloxacin as therapy for experimental osteomyelitis caused by *Pseudomonas aeruginosa*. J. Infect. Dis. 151(2): 291-294, 1985.

Norris, M.L. Gerbils. In: *UFAW Handbook on the Care and Management of Laboratory Animals,* 6th ed. T. Poole, ed. Churchill Livingstone Inc., New York, 1987.

Olson, M.E., and P. Renchko. Azaperone and azaperone-ketamine as a neuroleptic sedative and anesthetic in rats and mice. Lab. Anim. Sci. 38(3): 299-304, 1988.

O'Rourke, C.M., G.K. Peter, and P.L. Juneau. Evaluation of etamine-xylazine-acpromazine as a combination anesthetic regimen in mice. Contemp. Top. Lab. Anim. Sci. 33: A-25, 1994 (Abstract).

Page, C.D. Current reptilian anesthesia procedures. In: *Zoo & Wild Animal Medicine. Current Therapy 3.* M.E. Fowler, ed., 140-152. W.B. Saunders Company, Philadelphia, 1993.

Page, C.D., and M. Mautino. Clinical management of tortoises. Compend. Contin. Educ. Pract. Vet. 12(2): 221-230, 1990.

Papaioannou, V.E., and J.G. Fox. Efficacy of tribromoethanol anesthesia in mice. Lab. Anim. Sci. 43:189-192, 1993.

Patton, N.M. What every practitioner should know about rabbits and rodents. Calif. Vet. 33(5): 25-33, 1979.

Payton, A.J., and J.R. Pick. Evaluation of a combination of tiletamine and zolazepaqm as an anesthetic for ferrets. Lab. Anim. Sci. 39(3): 243-246, 1989.

Peardon, D.L., J.M. Tufts, and H.C. Eschenroeder. Experimental treatment of laboratory rats naturally infected with *Trichosomoides crassicauda.* Invest. Urol. 4: 215-219, 1966.

Pernikoff, D.S., and J. Orkin. Bacterial meningitis syndrome: An overall review of the disease complex and considerations of cross infectivity between great apes and man. In: *Proceedings of the Annual Meeting of the American Association of Zoo Veterinarians,* 235-241, 1991.

Perrin, A., G. Milano, A. Thyss, P. Cambon, and M. Schneider. Biochemical and pharmacological consequences of the interaction between methotrexate and ketoprofen in the rabbit. Br. J. Cancer 62:736-741, 1990.

Popilskis, S.J., M.C. Oz, P. Gorman, A. Florestal, and D.F. Kohn. Comparison of xylazine with tiletamine-zolazepam (Telazol) and xylazine-ketamine anesthesia in rabbits. Lab. Anim. Sci. 41: 51-53, 1991.

Post, K., and J.R. Saunders. Topical treatment of experimental ringworm in guinea pigs with griseofulvin in dimethylsulfoxide. Can. Vet. J. 20(2): 45-48, 1979.

Ralph, J., M.K. Stoskopf, and J.D. Strandberg. Serum gentamicin levels in baboons. Lab. Anim. Sci. 39(5): 475, 1989 (Abstract).

Raphael, B.L. Pet rabbit medicine. Compend. Contin. Educ. Pract. Vet. 3(1): 60-64, 1981.

Reiser, H.J., U.G. Whitworth, Jr., D.L. Hatchell, F.S. Sutherland, S. Nanda, T. McAdoo, and J.R. Hardin. Experimental diabetes in cats induced by partial pancreatectomy alone or combined with local injection of alloxan. Lab. Anim. Sci. 37(4): 449-452, 1987.

Reiss, C.S., J.M. Herrman, and R.E. Hopkins II. Effect of anthelminthic treatment on the immune response of mice. Lab. Anim. Sci. 37(6): 773-775, 1987.

Rettig, R., H. Stauss, C. Folberth, D. Ganten, R. Waldherr, and T. Unger. Hypertension transmitted by kidneys from stroke-prone spontaneously hypertensive rats. Am. J. Physiol. 257: F197-F203, 1989.

Richardson, V.C.G. Treatments. In: *Diseases of Domestic Guinea Pigs.* Blackwell Scientific Publications, Boston, 1992

Roach, P.D., P.M. Wallis, and M.E. Olson. The use of metronidazole, tinidazole and dimetridazole in eliminating trichomonads from laboratory mice. Lab. Anim. 22: 361-364, 1988.

Roman, R.J., and J.L. Osborn. Renal function and sodium balance in conscious Dahl S and R rats. Am. J. Physiol. 252: R833-R841, 1987.

Rosenberg, D.P. Nonhuman primate analgesia. Lab. Anim. 20:22, 1991.

Rosenberg, D.P., R.L. De Villez, and C.A. Gleiser. *Pemphigus vulgaris* in a baboon. Lab. Anim. Sci. 37(4): 489-491, 1987.

Rosskopf, W.J., Jr. Clinical use of selected therapeutics (Letter). J. Assoc. Avian Vet. 3(3): 127-128, 1989.

Rossoff, I.F. *Handbook of Veterinary Drugs.* Springer Publ. Co., Inc., New York, 1974.

Russell, R.J., D.K. Johnson, and J.A. Stunkard. *A Guide to Diagnosis, Treatment, and Husbandry of Pet Rabbits and Rodents.* Veterinary Medicine Publ., Edwardsville, KA, 1981.

Ryland, L.M., and J.R. Gorham. The ferret and its diseases. J. Am. Vet. Med. Assoc. 173(9): 1154-1158, 1978.

Sander, J.E. Basic information on guinea pigs. Vet. Forum (August): 28-29, 1992.

Sanders, E.A., R.D. Gleed, and P.W. Nathanielsz. Anesthetic management for instrumentation of the pregnant rhesus monkey. J. Med. Primatol. 20:223-228, 1991.

Schobert, E. Telazol® use in wild and exotic animals. Vet. Med. (October): 1080-1088, 1987.

Schofield, L.D., B.T. Bennett, W.E. Collins, and F.Z. Beluhan. An outbreak of *Plasmodium inui* in a colony of diabetic rhesus monkeys. Lab. Anim. Sci. 35(2): 167-168, 1985.

Schuchman, S.M. Individual care and treatment of rabbits, mice, rats, guinea pigs, hamsters, and gerbils, In: *Current Veterinary Therapy VI: Small Animal Practice.* R.W. Kirk, ed., 726-756. Saunders, Philadelphia, PA, 1977.

Schultz, C.S. *Formulary.* Veterinary Hospital Pharmacy, Washington State University, Washington State University Press, Pulman, WA, 1989.

Schumann, R.E., M.E. Harold, P.C. Gillette, M.M. Swindle, and C.H. Gaymes. Prophylactic treatment of swine with bretylium for experimental cardiac catherization. Lab. Anim. Sci. 43:244-246, 1993.

Sheffield, F.W., and E. Beveridge. Prophylaxis of "wet tail" in hamsters. Nature 196: 294-295, 1962.

Siegmund, O.H., ed. *The Merck Veterinary Manual,* 5th ed., 1979.

Silverman, J., M. Huhndorf, M. Balk, and G. Slater. Evaluation of a combination of tiletamine and zolazepam as an anesthetic for laboratory rodents. Lab. Anim. Sci. 33(5): 457-460, 1983.

Simmons, M.L., H.E. Williams, and E.B. Wright. Therapeutic value of the organic phosphate trichlorfon against *Syphacia obvelata* in inbred mice. Lab. Anim. Care 15(6): 382-385, 1965.

Smith, G.D., and T.G. Snider, III. Experimental infection and treatment of *Dentostomella translucida* in the Mongolian gerbil. Lab. Anim. Sci. 38(3): 339-340, 1988.

Snipes, K.P. *Pasteurella* in reptiles. In: *Diseases of Amphibians and Reptiles.* G.L. Hoff, F.L. Frye, and E.R. Jacobson, eds. Plenum Press, New York, 1984.

Strittmatter, J. Anaesthesie beim goldhamster mit ketamine und methoxyflurane. Z. Versuchstierk. Bd. 14: 129-133, 1972.

Strother, N.E., and W.S. Stokes. Evaluation of yohimbine and tolazoline as reversing agents for ketamine-xylazine anesthesia in the guinea pig. Lab. Anim. Sci. 39(5): 482, 1989 (Abstract).

Strunk, R.W., J.C. Gratz, R. Maserati, and W.M. Scheld. Comparison of ciprofloxacin with azlocillin plus tobramycin in the therapy of experimental *Pseudomonas aeruginosa* endocarditis. Antimicrob. Agents Chemother. 28: 428-432, 1985.

Summa, M.E.L., L. Ebisui, J.T. Osaka, and E.M.C. de Tolosa. Efficacy of oral ivermectin against *Trichosomoides crassicauda* in naturally infected laboratory rats. Lab. Anim. Sci. 42:620-622, 1992.

Sundlof, S. F., J.E. Riviere, and A.L. Craigmill. *Food Animal Residue Avoidance Databank Trade Name File. A Comprehensive Compendium of Food Animal Drugs,* 7th ed. Institute for Food and Agricultural Sciences, University of Florida, Gainesville.

Swindle, M.M., and R.J. Adams, eds. *Experimental Surgery and Physiology: Induced Animal Models of Human Disease.* Williams and Wilkens, Baltimore, MD, 1988.

Taber, R., and S. Irwin. Anesthesia in the mouse. Fed. Proc. 28(4): 1528-1532, 1969.

Takimoto, G., C. Jones, W. Lands, A. Bauman, J. Jeffrey, and O. Jonasson. Biochemical changes in rhesus monkey during the first days after streptozotocin administration are indicative of selective beta cell destruction. Metabolism 37(4): 364-370, 1988.

Taylor, D.M. Eradication of pinworms (*Syphacia obvelata*) from Syrian hamsters in quarantine. Lab. Anim. Sci. 42:413-414, 1992.

Thayer, C.B., S. Lowe, W.C. Rubright. Clinical evaluation of a combination of droperidol and fentanyl as an anesthetic for the rat and hamster. J. Am Vet. Med. Assoc. 161:665-668, 1972.

Trim, C.M., A. Palminteri, D.C. Sawyer, J.A.E. Hubbell, D.J. Krahwinkel, Jr., and K. Shaw. The use of oxymorphone in veterinary medicine. Proceedings of a roundtable. Veterinary Learning Systems Co., Inc., 1987.

Unay, E.S., and B.J. Davis. Treatment of *Syphacia obvelata* in the Syrian hamster (*Mesocricetus auratus*) with piperazine citrate. Am. J. Vet. Res. 41(11): 1899-1900, 1980.

United States Department of Agriculture. *Domestic Rabbits: Diseases and Para-*

sites, Agriculture Handbook, 490. Washington D.C., 1976.

University of Washington Regional Primate Research Center, Colony Division. Antibiotics routinely used for treatment, Seattle, 1987.

Van Riper, D.C., P.W. Day, J. Fineg, and J.R. Prine. Intestinal parasites of recently imported chimpanzees. Lab. Anim. Sci. 16(4): 360-363, 1966.

Wagner, J.E. Control of mouse pinworms, *Syphacia obvelata,* utilizing dichlorvos. Lab. Anim. Care 20(1): 39-44, 1970.

Waterman, A.E., and A. Livingston. Effects of age and sex on ketamine anesthesia in the rat. Br. J. Anesth. 50:885-888, 1978.

Wedemeyer, G. Stress of anesthesia with MS-222 and benzocaine in rainbow trout (*Salmo gairdneri*). J. Fish. Res. Board Can. 27: 909, 1970.

Weihe, W.H. The laboratory rat. In: *UFAW Handbook on the Care and Management of Laboratory Animals,* 6th ed. T. Poole, ed. Churchill Livingstone Inc., New York, 1987.

Weisbroth, S.H., and J.H. Fudens. Use of ketamine hydrochloride as an anesthetic in laboratory rabbits, rats, mice, and guinea pigs. Lab. Anim. Sci. 22(6): 904-906, 1972.

Weisbroth, S.H., and S. Scher. *Trichosomoides crassicauda* infection of a commercial rat breeding colony. 2. Drug screening for anthelmintic activity and field trials with methyridine. Lab. Anim. Sci. 21(2): 213-219, 1971.

Welch, W.D., Y-S. Lu, and R.E. Bawdon. Pharmacokinetics of penicillin-G in serum and nasal washings of *Pasteurella multocida* free and infected rabbits. Lab. Anim. Sci. 37(1): 65-68, 1987.

Welshman, M.D. Management of newly imported primates. Anim. Tech. 36(2): 125-129, 1985.

Whitney, R. Hamsters. In: *Animals for Research: Principles of Breeding and Management.* W. Lane-Petter, ed., 365-392. Academic Press, New York, 1963.

Whitney, R.A., Jr., D.J. Johnson, and W.C. Cole. *Laboratory Primate Handbook.* Academic Press, New York, 1973.

Whitney, R.A., Jr., J.B. Mulder, and D.K. Johnson. Nonhuman primates: Bacterial diseases. In: *Nonhuman Primates.* ACLAM Laboratory Animal Medicine and Science Series. G.L. Van Hoosier, Jr., coord., 77-94. University of Washington, Seattle, WA, 1977.

Wilhelmi, G. Species differences in susceptibility to the gastro-ulcerogenic action of anti-inflammatory agents. Parmacology 11:220-230, 1974.

Williams, C.S.F. *Practical Guide to Laboratory Animals.* C.V. Mosby, St. Louis, MO, 1976.

Williams, C.S.F. Guinea pigs and rabbits. Small Anim. Pract. 9(3): 487-497, 1979.

Wing, S.R., C.H. Courtney, and M.D. Young. Effect of ivermectin on murine mites. J. Am. Vet. Med. Assoc. 187(11): 1191-1192, 1985.

Wissman, M., and B. Parsons. Surgical removal of a lipoma-like mass in a lemur (*Lemur fulvus fulvus*). J. Small Exotic Anim. Med. 2:8-12, 1992.

Wixson, S.K. Anesthesia and analgesia. In: *The Biology of the Laboratory Rabbit,* 2nd edition. P.J. Manning, D.H. Ringler, and C.E. Newcomer, eds., 87-109. Academic Press, New York, 1994.

Wixson, S.K., W.J. White, H.C. Hughes, Jr., C.M. Lang, and W.K. Marshall. A comparison of pentobarbital, fentanyl-droperidol, ketamine-xylazine and ketamine-diazepam anesthesia in adult male rats. Lab. Anim. Sci. 37(6): 726-730, 1987.

Wright, E.M., K.L. Marcella, J.F. Woodson. Animal pain: Evaluation and control. Lab. Anim. 14:20-36, 1985.

Wolf, R.H., S.V. Gibson, E.A. Watson, and G.B. Baskin. Multidrug chemotherapy of tuberculosis in rhesus monkeys. Lab. Anim. Sci. 38(1): 25-33, 1988.

Wolff, P.L. The parasites of New World primates: A review. In: Proceedings of the annual meeting of tyhe American Association of Zoo Veterinarians, 87-94, 1990.

Young, J.D., W.J. Hurst, W.J. White, and C.M. Lang. An evaluation of ampicillin pharmacokinetics and toxicity in guinea pigs. Lab. Anim. Sci. 37(5): 652-656, 1987.

Zajac, A., J.F. Williams, and C.S.F. Williams. Mange caused by *Trixacarus caviae* in guinea pigs. J. Am. Vet. Med. Assoc. 177(9): 900-903, 1980.

INDEX

ISBN 0-8138-2422-2

9 780813 824222

90000>

Iowa State University Press
2121 South State Avenue
Ames, IA 50014

Phone: 800-862-6657
Fax: 515-292-3348